Spirituality and Nursing Practice

JUDY HARRISON
PHILIP BURNARD

Avebury

Aldershot · Brookfield USA · Hong Kong · Singapore · Sydney

Published by
Avebury
Ashgate Publishing Limited
Gower House
Croft Road
Aldershot
Hants GU11 3HR
England

Ashgate Publishing Company
Old Post Road
Brookfield
Vermont 05036
USA

British Library Cataloguing in Publication Data

Harrison, Judy
    Spirituality and Nursing Practice
    I. Title II. Burnard, Philip
    362.1

ISBN 1 85628 509 X

Printed and Bound in Great Britain by
Athenaeum Press Ltd, Newcastle upon Tyne.

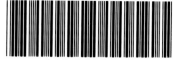

DATE DUE

Demco No. 62-0549

SPIRITUALITY AND NURSING PRACTICE

For Susie and Norman
and for Sally, Aaron and Rebecca

Contents

Acknowledgements

There are a number of people to whom Judy owes a great deal of gratitude, indeed, without them her contribution to this book would not have been possible. First, grateful thanks to the trained members of nursing staff and the non-nurses who shared so openly so much of themselves and their experiences. Second, thanks are extended to Barbara Pepworth, Margaret Bawn and Jo Wilkins for transcribing the interviews and for their secretarial support. Thanks also go to the management of the Avon and Gloustershire College of Health, Bristol for all their support. Finally, grateful thanks to Judy's family, friends, colleagues, students and patients for their continued encouragement, enthusiasm, patience and inspiration.

As always, Philip would like to thank his wife Sally for all her love and support and his children, Aaron and Rebecca for their love and patience.

Introduction

Increasingly, nursing is referred to as being concerned with holistic care. This usually means that it is thought that nurses should do more than simply look after patients' and clients' physical needs. They should also care for the psychological, social and spiritual aspects of the person. Yet if we consider each of these in turn, we may find that things are not so straightforward. Clearly, the physical domain is the one that is most straightforward and perhaps easiest to consider. Physical care involves consideration of the concrete fact of another person's anatomy, physiology and pathology. Psychological needs have also been well mapped out and while the psychological domain is not as clear cut as the physical, there is a considerable psychological tradition in the caring professions. Similarly, sociology offers considerable insights into how nurses might consider patients' and clients' social needs. Perhaps the most difficult dimension of care is the *spiritual* dimension. Variously described as involving acts of faith and belief, being of a 'personal nature' and generally being thought of as part of the metaphysical, the spiritual domain is not always easy to talk about or define. Further, while it may be possible to identify nursing strategies that consider people's physical, psychological and social needs, trying to identify the parameters of spiritual care is problematic.

It is with these factors in mind that the study reported here was designed. The study was a qualitative, descriptive study of trained nurses' perceptions of spirituality from both personal and professional points of view. Spirituality in nursing appears to be a complex yet significant aspect of nursing and this study explored trained nurses' perceptions of such a concept in order to begin to map out the territory. In addition, the findings of the study helped in the development of a tentative theoretical and practical model for practice in nursing and enabled the researchers to develop educational principles in this fraught area.

The book offers a start in the ground-clearing process of exploring what spiritual care in nursing might mean. It offers a review of some of the literature on spirituality in nursing, the results of a qualitative and descriptive study into the topic and some indications of how spirituality can be addressed in nurse education. It is hoped that it will provide ideas and inspiration for other researchers and educators who are finding their own way in this difficult but crucial field.

1 Spirituality

Often linked to the idea of religion, spirituality is a broad and diverse concept that has been defined and discussed in many different ways. While it is often linked with religion, that link is by no means a necessity when exploring the concept. This chapter examines a variety of aspects of spirituality, from various perspectives. In order to begin to appreciate and understand the concept of spirituality as it applies to nursing, four different approaches have been taken: definitions of spirituality, spiritual needs, spiritual well-being, and spiritual distress.

Definitions of spirituality

It appears that the nursing literature refers to the totality of the person as encompassing body, mind and spirit (Belcher et al 1989, Bowers 1987, Labun 1988). Whereas it could be stated that body refers to the physiological elements of the person and mind the psychological and emotional elements, it is less clear what is meant by spirit.

Kreidler cited by Labun (1988) in her study of the nursing literature, found in most cases the word spirituality is often equated or used synonymously with the word religion. Peterson (1985) notes that generally religion is used to describe an organised set of beliefs and practices expressing and representing those beliefs. However it would appear that spirituality can be defined in broader terms and refers to a complex area of human experience.

From an anthropological point of view, Geertz (1966) defined religion thus:

> Without further ado, then, a *religion* is: 1) a system of symbols which acts to 2) establish powerful, pervasive and long-lasting moods and motivations in men by 3) formulating conceptions of a general order of existence and 4) clothing these conceptions with such an aura of factuality that 5) the moods and motivations seem uniquely realistic.

Clearly, Geertz' analysis was a critical one and, following Durkheim, Weber and Freud, he saw religion as a cultural system. His framework, summarised above allowed him to offer a detailed and broad ranging analysis of religious experience. Jung, in a different and more psychological sense, also took a broad view of the idea of religion:

> Religion appears to me to be a peculiar attitude of mind which could be formulated in accordance with the original use of the word *religion*, which means a careful consideration and observation of certain dynamic factors that are conceived as 'powers': spirits, daemons, gods, laws, ideals, or whatever name man has given to such factors in his world as he has found powerful, dangerous, or helpful enough to be taken into careful consideration, or grand, beautiful, and meaningful enough to be devoutly worshipped and loved. (Jung 1961).

It is notable that neither of these two authors necessarily saw God as a central focus of the idea of the religious. Indeed, in an earlier section of his book *Psychology and Religion*, Jung summarised his definition of the concept thus:

> In speaking of religion I must make clear from the start what I mean by that term. Religion, as the Latin word denotes, is a careful and scrupulous observation of what Rudolf Otto aptly termed the *numinosum*, that is, a dynamic agency or effect not caused by an arbitrary act of will. On the contrary, it seizes and controls the human subject, who is always rather its victim than its creator. (Jung 1961).

5

Whilst Jung seemed to make the concept of religion 'larger' than just a question of a set of religions beliefs, it is also notable that in his definition, above, he writes of the passivity of the individual and of a religious experience 'seizing the human subject' who is 'not the creator' of the act. Jung's sense of mystery and of the numinous was captured well by the 16th century mystic, Jakob Boehme, in his book *The Signature of All Things*:

All whatever is taught of God, without the knowledge of the signature is dumb and void of understanding; for it proceeds only from an historical conjecture, from the mouth of another, wherein the spirit without knowledge is dumb; but as the spirit opens to him the *signature*, then he understands the speech of another; and further, he understands how the spirit has manifested and revealed itself (out of the essence through the principle) in the sound of the voice. For though I see one to speak, teach, preach, and write of God, and though I hear and read the same, yet this is not sufficient for me to understand him; but if his sound and spirit out of his signature and similitude enter into my own similitude and imprint his similitude into mine, then I may understand him really and fundamentally, be it either spoken or written, if he has the hammer that can strike my bell...(Boehme translated by Law 1781).

In this passage, Boehme, so many centuries ago, seems to capture many of the issues that are relevant in this study and in modern concepts of spirituality and care. His words seem to suggest that there must be a 'signature' - a key to understanding, that once discovered, can make words and abstractions 'real'. Boehme also seems to hint at a much later concept of *empathy* in this passage - 'if he has the hammer that can strike my bell...'. We shall see, also, that a number of respondents in the current study referred to the idea of 'becoming aware of God' or suggested metaphors of 'doors opening' as images of understanding, of revelation and realisation. Boehme also seems to be suggesting that knowledge of God is 'special' knowledge: it is necessary to have the 'key' (or the signature) in order to know something of God.

In passing, it is also worth noting that by the early 1960's there was a considerable debate about the notion of religion without a formal sense of 'God up there or God out there' (Robinson 1963) - the notorious 'Honest to God debate. Earlier, Paul Tillich had described the idea of God in terms of the 'ground of our being' and his definition is worth quoting at length because it links, well, to our discussion on the nature of spirituality in nursing:

> The name of this infinite and inexhaustible depth and ground of all being is *God*. That depth is what the word *God* means. And if that word has not much meaning for you, translate it, and speak of the depths of your life, of the source of your being, or your ultimate concern, of what you take seriously without any reservation. Perhaps, in order to do so, you must forget everything traditional that you have learned about God, perhaps even that word itself. For if you know that God means depth, you know much about him. You cannot then call yourself an atheist or unbeliever. For you cannot think or say: Life has no depth! Life is shallow. Being itself is surface only. If you could say this in complete seriousness, you would be an atheist; but otherwise you are not. He who knows about depth knows about God (Tillich 1949).

God, for Tillich, cannot be located 'above' the world, for 'above' only exists when a 'flat-earth' view is held. There can be no 'up there' in our present view of the universe. Instead, Tillich suggests that God is, almost in contradiction to traditional thinking, 'depth'. But the depth of which Tillich talks is not a depth in some sort of universal geography but a *human* depth: a depth of experience and feeling, perhaps. Tillich's depth is almost a *psychological* depth, although the word seems inadequate. It is intriguing to note that Boehme also referred to 'the great Deep of this World' (Boehme 1954), thus anticipating Tillich by some 400 years.

Already, then, the picture is complicated: spirituality is sometimes used synonymously with religion and religion may or may not incorporate traditional views of God. As we shall see in other chapters, how God and religion are defined also relates very much to the particular *faith* that is held and is often linked to culture.

Spirituality has been described as, a belief that relates a person to the world, giving meaning to existence (Soeken and Carson 1987); the central philosophy of life which guides peoples conduct (Ellerhorst-Ryan 1985); a force that impels humans forward into living (Bugental and Bugental 1984); a personal quest to find meaning and purpose in life (Burkhardt and Nagai-Jacobson 1985, Granstrom 1985); and a transcendental relationship or

7

sense of connection with mystery, a Higher Being, God[1] or Universe (Ellis 1980, O'Brien 1982). It would seem that spirituality within these definitions could refer to religion but could also include more philosophical ideas of belief and meaning in life.

Lane (1987) explains that the spiritual dimension manifests itself in four ways. Transcending, which is the desire to step beyond who and what people are, aspiring to be something and know something more, to love more and create more; connecting and belonging, the desire to belong to someone, something, somewhere; giving life, the desire to give to others, to make life better; and finally Being Free, the desire to have and seek choices, to exercise options.

Fish and Shelly, cited by Peterson (1985), suggest that the spiritual component involves three aspects. Firstly, it imports a sense of meaning and purpose in life, which may help to answer or tolerate lack of answers to some of the questions that accompany life experiences eg: "why is this happening to me?". Secondly it provides a means of forgiveness, without which individuals may be forced to live with their imperfections and failures and which therefore provide a way to solve such questions as "what did I do to deserve this?". Finally it is a source of love and relatedness, perhaps the only defence against the inevitable times of aloneness and abandonment even when surrounded by others, so providing a sense of dignity and worth.

Thus, spirituality can be considered a conscious or unconscious belief that relates individuals to the world and gives meaning and definition to existence. As Granstrom (1985) notes, it is the spiritual dimension of human beings that is life giving and integrating. It is the spirit that makes humans more than the material reality in which they are surrounded, as well as what makes humans unique from any other material being (Lane 1987).

Spiritual needs

Hess and Stoll, cited by Ellerhorst-Ryan (1985), two nurses who are well known for their interest in the spiritual concerns of patients, have defined spiritual needs as factors necessary to establish and maintain a relationship with God - however God is defined by the individuals. Nevertheless, in keeping with the more broadly defined concept of spirituality, O'Brien (1982)

---

[1] God will be referred to in the masculine form throughout this book.

8

identifies spiritual needs as:

> ... involving any essential variables required for the support and viability of that element which inspires in man the desire to transcend the realm of the material world. (O'Brien 1982)

Perhaps the simpler explanation given by Bollinger cited by Peterson (1985) is easier to understand, where spiritual needs are seen as the deepest requirements of the self. If met they make it possible for people to function with meaningful identity and purpose, so that in all stages of life they may relate to reality with hope. Indeed Bugental and Bugental (1984) suggest that this need to make sense of one's life in terms of some kind of meaning is a basic human need.

Hess and Stoll, cited by Ellerhorst-Ryan (1985), identified specific spiritual needs which included forgiveness, love, hope, trust and meaning and purpose in life. The 5th National Conference on Nursing Diagnosis supported this approach by incorporating the five spiritual needs into the Spiritual Distress Diagnostic Category (Kim and Moritz 1980). In addition Highfield and Cason (1983) used a spiritual needs approach in their investigation as to whether surgical nurses caring for oncology patients were aware of patients' spiritual concerns. These needs were identified as, the need for meaning and purpose in life, the need to receive love, the need to give love and the need for hope and creativity.

Nevertheless, although these spiritual needs are present, it appears they develop and find expression in different ways. The qualities of forgiveness and love can be experienced in relationships between people, as well as relying on an existing philosophy of life and or belief system (Peterson 1985). As Labun (1988) states, it is relationships such as these that can bring meaning and fulfilment to life, providing a purpose.

On the other hand, meaning may be found through adherence to an existing ideological view point be it physiological, psychological, sociological or political. Others take the view that there is no meaning to life except that which is invested into it by the individuals themselves (Kopp 1974) and those with a particular positivistic scientific view of the world may dismiss the metaphysical altogether and thus the notion of a spiritual problem does not arise for them (Burnard 1987).

It may be that these needs are significantly influenced by an ethnic or cultural background where spiritual needs are met through a set of cultural practices (O'Brien 1982). Yet another vehicle for the expression is institutionalised religion. As Labun (1988) notes, spiritual needs are channelled through such avenues as prayers, rituals, and worship. It provides meaning in day to day living and helps people through personal hardship such as pain, illness and personal disaster. In addition it provides an avenue for celebration when hardships are overcome. Labun (1988) also identifies meaningful, purposeful or creative work as an expression of spirituality and points out that work as a service to mankind may fulfil spiritual needs as may writing, for example poetry.

Spiritual well being

Byrne (1985) reports that at the White House Conference in 1981, spiritual well being was defined as:

> ... the affirmation of life in a relationship with God, self, community and environment that nurtures and celebrates wholeness (Byrne 1985).

Wholeness is emphasised in contrast to fragmentation and isolation. This definition appears to comprise of both a religious and sociopsychological component, which could be described as vertical and horizontal dimensions. The vertical dimension refers to the sense of well being in the relationship with God, as defined by the individual, while the horizontal refers to a sense of purpose in and satisfaction with life (Ellerhorst-Ryan 1985, Stoll 1989).

However, Ellison cited by Stoll (1989) contends that spiritual well being is not a state but an indication of the presence of spiritual health in a person. Thus spiritual well being is defined as behavioural expressions of spiritual health, eg. feeling life is a positive experience, feeling fulfilled and satisfied with life, feeling a sense of inner harmony. Highfield and Cason (1983) outline signs of spiritual health using a needs based framework and give similar examples of behaviour. Their framework is illustrated in Figure 1.1. It could therefore be argued that spiritual well being or integrity could be present when people experience wholeness within themselves, with other human beings, or in transcendence with another realm. This could be likened to what Maslow (1970) has described as a 'peak experience', the opposite to that described by Frankl (1964) as an 'existential vacuum' characterised by despair, distress and a feeling of emptiness.

Need	Behaviour of Condition
Need for meaning and purpose in life	Expresses that he has lived in accordance with his value system in the past. Expresses desire to participate in religious rituals. Lives in accordance with his value system at present. Expresses contentment with his life. Expresses hope in future.
Need to receive love	Expresses hope in life after death. Expresses confidence in the health care team. Expresses feelings of being loved by others/God. Expresses feelings of forgiveness by others/God. Expresses desire to perform religious rituals leading to salvation. Trusts others/God with the outcome of a situation in which he feels he has no control.
Need to give love	Expresses love for others through actions. Seeks the good of others.
Need for hope and creativity	Asks for information about his condition realistically. Talks about his condition realistically. Sets realistic personal health goals. Uses time during illness/hospitalisation constructively. Values his inner self more than his physical self.

Figure 1.1 Signs of spiritual health (Highfield and Cason 1983, p.189)

Spiritual distress

Spiritual distress, dispiritedness, spiritual collapse and spiritual problems are all terms used by authors to convey altered spiritual integrity (Highfield and Cason 1983, Bugental and Bugental 1984, Burnard 1987, Stoll 1989, Belcher et al 1989).

Highfield and Cason (1983) identify signs of spiritual problems using a needs based framework and O'Brien (1982) has listed seven common human experiences under the category of altered spiritual integrity. These experiences include spiritual pain, alienation, anxiety, guilt, anger, loss and despair.

Spiritual distress is also a nursing diagnosis approved by the North American Nursing Diagnoses Association who provide further clarification of the term by identifying defining characteristics which include a variety of behaviours (Stoll 1989). For example, alteration of behaviour or mood evidenced by anger, crying, withdrawal, preoccupation, anxiety, hostility or apathy and questioning the meaning of existence and suffering. However the critical defining characteristic is expressing concern with the meaning of life/death or any belief system.

Spiritual distress therefore, may happen to those who are faced with some sort of extreme challenge in life and are left questioning the reason for such an occurrence eg. illness, bereavement, broken relationships. In psychological literature, Jung describes the problem of individuation (Storr 1983), as the quest for finding and understanding the self, which may be preceded by a feeling of pointlessness and lack of ability to be self motivated, the existential vacuum described by Frankl (1963).

Questions relating to meaning may also occur during particular stages in life (Carson 1989b), eg. the identity crisis of adolescence and early to middle age, when a person may reappraise and re-evaluate his/her own life. These may occur despite the fact that the person may hold well defined religious beliefs. Carson offers guidelines (Figure 1.2) for spiritual assessment.

The need to find meaning in what we do is very strong. It is probably the case that all human beings have to find meaning or face the problem of becoming dispirited. The question is often raised as to why certain things happen to us in the way that they do. This quest for meaning often becomes more acute in times of specific (and sometimes life-threatening) difficulty. The health professional often has to help people who are working through life-crises. The mere fact of being with people in this way can raise questions of meaning for the carer. The fact of being involved in other people's crises can also raise questions of meaning. The health professional who has to face the death of a client may well be tempted to raise the same sorts of 'why?' questions as did the client.

Nonverbal behaviour	1. Observe affect. Does the client's affect or attitude convey loneliness, depression, anger, agitation, or anxiety? 2. Observe behaviour. Does the client pray during the day? Does the client rely on religious reading material or other literature for solace?
Verbal behaviour	1. Does the client seem to complain out of proportion to his illness? 2. Does the client complain of sleeping difficulties? 3. Does the client ask for unusually high doses of sedation or pain medication? 4. Does the client refer to God in any way? 5. Does the client talk about prayer, faith, hope, or anything of a religious nature? 6. Does the client talk about church functions that are a part of his life? 7. Does the client express concern over the meaning and direction of life? Does the client express concern over the impact of the illness on the meaning of life?
Interpersonal relationships	1. Does the client have visitors or does he spend visiting hours alone? 2. Are the visitors supportive or do they seem to leave the client feeling upset? 3. Does the client have visitors from his church? 4. Does the client interact with the staff and other clients?
Environment	1. Does the client have a Bible or other religious reading material with him? 2. Does the client wear religious medals or pins? 3. Does the client use religious articles such as statues in observing religious practices? 4. Has the client received religious get-well cards? 5. Does the client use personal pictures, artwork, or music to keep his spirits up

Figure 1.2 Guidelines for spiritual assessment (after Carson 1989, p.158)

Helping other people to find meaning and searching for meaning ourselves can both be stressful activities. Finding a framework for making sense of life can also be problematic. Such frameworks often manifest themselves in very different sorts of ways. For some, a set of religious precepts helps in the process of making sense of life. For others, a philosophical, political or psychological set of beliefs and values is what helps to add meaning.

Perhaps the most stressful situation of all is the fact of having an inability to find meaning at all. Such a state may be described as *dispiritedness.*

13

Dispiritedness, then, is the fact of being unable to invest life with meaning. It is sometimes, but not always, combined with depression. When it is not, it is characterised by a general sense of loss, a lack of conviction in what one is doing and a lack of enthusiasm for life in general. It may also be accompanied by a sense of cynicism and by the development of 'gallows humour'.

Some commentators have gone further and formally defined the notion of spiritual distress. Kim, McFarland, and McLane (1987) define spiritual distress as:

> ...distress of the human spirit...a disruption in the life principle which pervades a person's entire being and which integrates and transcends one's biological and psychosocial nature.

It may be argued, in passing, that the first part of this definition is tautological and that the second raises questions about what we are to understand by the idea of 'the life principle'. Kim, McFarland and McLane go on to offer defining characteristics of spiritual distress. These are:

- Expresses concern with meaning of life/death or any belief system
- Anger towards God
- Questions meaning of suffering
- Verbalises inner conflict about beliefs
- Verbalises concern about relationships with deity
- Questions meaning of own existence
- Unable to participate in usual religious practices
- Seeks spiritual assistance
- Questions moral or ethical implications of therapeutic regimen
- Gallows humour
- Displacement of anger toward religious representatives
- Nightmares of sleep disturbance
- Alteration of behaviour or mood evidenced by anger, crying, withdrawal, preoccupation, anxiety, hostility or apathy (Kim, McFarland and McLane 1987).

This notion of spiritual distress appears to suggest that it is something that may occur in those who have previously held religious beliefs and who are now questioning them. It is suggested here that the notion of spiritual distress may be better conceptualised as a concern with ultimate things and with

14

meaning. In this way, it is quite possible to argue that atheists and agnostics are just as capable of experiencing spiritual distress as are those who have, or who have had, religious convictions (Burnard 1988). Spiritual distress, in these terms, is characterised more than anything else by a profound sense of meaninglessness. This sense of meaninglessness is well described in the literature. Sartre's hero (or anti-hero) in *Nausea* experiences that feeling. He finds himself caught up in the world but not really part of it. He notices himself observing others but not being moved by them. In fact he is rarely moved by anything. Instead he experiences a profound sense of isolation and distaste for life. Such a position is one that Hesse's character, Harry Haller, in *Steppenwolf* is familiar with. Aware of a 'darker' side to his personality, Haller also feels himself to be an observer of life rather than a participant in it. What is notable, though, is that Haller can *live* with his situation. Rather than being totally overcome by it, he copes and he continues to live. It seems likely that there are many people who find themselves living meaningless lives but nevertheless cope. We should not, necessarily take the view that meaninglessness is pathological and that somehow 'something must be done about it'. For some, it would seems, it becomes a way of life.

Sometimes, such meaninglessness comes as a result of working in situations that are demanding of our emotions. The processes of caring for others, of listening to other people's problems and of having to be altruistic all take their toll. We cannot expect to continue to give to others without at some point feeling a sense of being 'used up'. Unfortunately, as we have noted, the health professions are not, generally, very good at supporting each other. Thus it is quite possible to be in a caring role and have continual demands made on one's time and resources without anyone else attempting to lift the load. In time, it is possible to reach a state of meaninglessness through sheer emotional (and possibly, spiritual) exhaustion.

Aloneness

One of the corollaries of dispiritedness is a sense of aloneness that can accompany it. Sometimes, however, an aloneness can arise out of a person's life philosophy. Sartre (1948), perhaps the best know exponent of the type of philosophising known as existentialism acknowledge's the *aloneness* of the individual. He notes that, as author's of our own existence we are both free and responsible. Clearly, the two go together. It would be difficult to argue that we were free and yet *not* responsible. The notion of freedom is

15

inextricably bound up with responsibility. In being free and responsible, Sartre's person is also alone in his decision making. No one can decide for him: he alone can make decisions for himself for this is part of what it means to be free and responsible. Whilst this seems to be *literally* true, in that, in the end, we do have to choose for ourselves, Sartre's position seems to discount the fact that we live alongside other people. Whilst our final act of decision making may be our own, in the process of reaching that decision, we are invariably advised by others. Sartre argues that it is only trivial decisions that are 'decided for us'. He cites, as an example, the choice of whether or not to have a cake with your coffee (Sartre 1964).

On the other hand, a little reflection may reveal that many of the much larger decisions that we make are also made in conjunction with other people. Before I move house, or job or get married, I invariably discuss these decisions with others and are to a greater or lesser degree influenced by them. It seems almost a trivial point to say that, despite that influence, we still chose *alone*. The final choice may be ours but the process of making the decision has been a joint one. Aloneness may be a product of existentialism, itself, for the fact that it focuses so extensively on the individual may account, in part, for the existentialist feeling cut off from other people. It is notable, for example, how often other people are *rejected* by existential writers. Sartre's hero, in his novel, *Nausea*, for example, distances himself from others seemingly by choice. To distance yourself from others seems like a reasonable recipe for aloneness. Colin Wilson's analysis of 'the outsider' in literature is full of references to other existential heros who cut themselves off from other people (Wilson 1956). In such cases, aloneness may or may not be part of the syndrome that we have described as dispiritedness.

Intuition

Yet another aspect of spirituality is intuition - possibly one of the most difficult aspects to define. Intuition is one of the fundamental qualities of being a nurse. Frequently denied but often used, this quality or characteristic is one that can help us to understand our patients, our colleagues and ourselves.

What is intuition? Jung maintained that the mind has a least four functions (Jung 1983): thinking, feeling, sensing and intuiting. Most of us are familiar with the first two. Sensing refers to our appreciation of the functioning of the senses: seeing, hearing, touching, tasting and smelling. We are often dependent on our senses for understanding what is going on around us. It is even possible to argue that we can *only* understand the world through references to our senses. Indeed, most of what we know and understand comes to us through one of the five special senses: we either read or see things; we are told or hear things; we feel things, taste or smell things.

Intuition, on the other hand, is knowledge *beyond* the senses. It is, for want of a better term: a 'sixth sense'. Stronger than suggestion or belief, we can arguably *know* via our intuitive ability. If we consider some of the important decisions we have made (inside and outside of nursing), many of them were made intuitively. One of the present authors can remember working with a Sister in the accident and emergency unit who looked and listened to a patient who was fully conscious and talking and who decided to make a 'crash call': a call for the cardiac arrest team. She 'knew' that he was about to arrest. And so he did. When asked, afterwards, how she could have known that he was about to arrest, she was unable to answer. Her experience, knowledge and, arguably, her intuition, had allowed her to make an irrational decision which proved to be lifesaving.

Nurses rely on an intuitive sense. We intuit when we go and have a second look at a patient in a ward. We use intuition when we ask particular sorts of questions when we are counselling patients (Burnard 1989). We also use intuition when we talk to colleagues and friends. We often know just the right question to ask at what seems to be exactly the wrong time. Arguably, again, we are combining a range of experience and knowledge with that far less tangible quality - intuition.

Carl Rogers, founder of client-centred therapy and counselling often described his intuitive sense at work in his therapy (Rogers 1967, 1980). He suggested that he was least happy with his work when he found himself using 'techniques' and was far happier when he acknowledged hunches and hidden feelings that he had. He came to realise that in following his intuition he was likely to help the client far more than if he stuck to the more logical approach. And perhaps this is true for many of us as nurses, tutors and friends. Whilst the logical approach clearly has its place, so does acting 'by the seat of our pants'.

And yet intuition has had something of a bad press. Why should this be the case? Perhaps it is because, in this culture, we have come to hold in high regard the positivistic or scientific approach. And rightly so. When researchers do research, we want to know that their methods are sound and valid. This is equally as true of qualitative research as it is of quantitative research. Qualitative research can never be a case of 'anything goes'. The qualitative researcher must be able to account for her findings and for her methods of analysis.

Unfortunately, this quest for validity has sometimes led to a sort of 'dustbowl' approach to research. Some researchers, both within nursing and without, are so taken with the idea of quantification and with validity, that they discount the notion of intuition as somehow 'unscientific'. It cannot easily be accounted for so it is best left alone. Yet most researchers, whatever their persuasion, depend to some degree on 'serendipity' or on chance findings. Doing research would indeed be dull if nothing happened that could not be accounted for!

There is another problem with intuition. A double edged form of sexism may be noted. On the one hand, the expression 'women's intuition' is often used to suggest that women may be more intuitive than men. This idea seems also to be encouraged by the psychologist Jung (1983) who argued that women tended to be more intuitive than men. This may lead to the belief that men are not intuitive or that they should not be. Unfortunately, too, given the fact that women are sometimes discriminated against in our society, there may be a tacit suggestion that rationality is somehow 'better' than intuition. This is certainly encouraged by our Western educational system which tends to prize rationality highly. All of these rather curious notions may have lead to a devaluing of intuition.

Thus it is argued, that intuition forms an important aspect of who we are and what we do. To *cultivate* intuition is the next step. If we have it, then perhaps we should *use* it. How, then do we cultivate it? Surely such a proposition is meaningless? By definition, intuition cannot easily be accounted for. How, then, are we to develop it? First, perhaps, we can acknowledge its existence. We can stay open to the idea of experiencing intuitive thoughts and feelings. We can trust our judgement and allow ourselves to take some risks in disclosing some of our intuitions to others. As we noted above, Carl Rogers was happiest when he worked in this way, in counselling. If we find that our intuitions turn out to be right, then we can come to respect our intuition even more. This is not an injunction to abandon logical and rational thought. Nursing is dependent upon such rationality. It is also dependent upon intuition, especially when the expert practitioner is at work (Benner 1984). The expert nurse often thinks and acts intuitively.

Second, we can be on the look out for what Jung called 'synchronicity' or meaningful coincidence. What is to be understood by 'meaningful coincidence'? Not *all* coincidence is particularly meaningful. On the other hand, many things appear to 'happen together', which *do* seem to make sense. We think of a friend and they phone us. We are talking about a patient and they walk through the door - and so on. If we allow ourselves to take notice of this synchronicity, we can allow ourselves to make links that can guide us to better practice. Such synchronicity often happens in counselling. The counsellor is thinking of something seemingly unattached to what is happening in the counselling relationship and the client begins to talk of that very thing. The nurse-as-counsellor can often become more skilled by leaving herself open to the idea of synchronicity.

Intuition will not stand on its own as a method of developing skills in nursing. If it is acknowledged and listened to, it can make the difference between the skilled nurse and the skilled and *human* nurse. For it is intuition which taps into that which is truly human - the part of us that makes it possible for us to truly care for another person. Arguably, the spiritual domain involves 'listening' to our intuitions as well as to the more rational side or ourselves.

Summary

Examination of these terms has allowed clarification of different facets of spirituality but it is not the total picture. As Stoll (1989) notes spirituality is multidimensional and complex. It is uniquely experienced and interpreted by each person and each person alone can provide another with unique perceptions of his/her own spirituality.

Yet it appears that spirituality is an important aspect of individuals, which provides meaningfulness and purpose in life, so creating a sense of wholeness or fulfilment. In addition spiritual needs can be expressed in different ways and it seems that for only some, does institutionalised religion act as a framework through which these needs can be met.

However it is important to note that one of the greatest problems about defining and discussing spirituality is that it is resistant to language. Rowan (1990) highlights the difficulties of explaining such basic matters as the colour red, or taste of strawberries or sexual passion to someone who has not experienced these things. To explain 'peak experience' or 'the meeting of a deeper self' or 'the vision of God' is hard to do in words and words can never be enough. Rowan (1990) suggests that this is because the transpersonal, by its very nature, goes beyond the neat boundaries that formal logic inevitably sets up. It is necessary to bear this in mind throughout any discussion of spirituality.

2 Beliefs and values

A belief has been described as a type of attitude (Tschudin 1986) and also as a conviction of the truth of some statement, especially when well grounded but not proven or tested empirically (Carson 1989a). Yet it appears that the beliefs of individuals will play a large part in determining their spiritual integrity as will values, faith and hope.

Religious beliefs

It would seem that most people need to make sense of their lives in terms of some kinds of meaning. Whilst some invest that meaning through a religious framework , there appears to be an absence of a generally accepted definition of religion. McGilloway (1985a) offers several. For example, people's relationship with a power, usually termed God; a way of living or a way of believing. Haralambos (1980) also reviews the many definitions but concludes that all tend to emphasise certain aspects of religion and yet exclude others, whether it be the nature of the religious belief itself or the religious practices.

However, Haralambos (1980) also notes that whilst the functionalist perspective emphasises the positive contributions of religion to society, it sometimes ignores the dysfunctional aspects. It tends to be preoccupied with harmony and integration and neglects the many instances where religion is a disruptive force. It bypasses the many examples of internal divisions within a community which have occurred over questions of religious worship and dogma eg. Northern Ireland and the Middle East. Nevertheless for the purpose of this study, religion is used to describe an organised set of beliefs and practices expressing or representing those beliefs which may help some individuals answer basic questions about life and death and the unexplained happenings of the world around (Peterson 1985).

McGilloway (1985a) notes that each religion has its own basic traditions, beliefs and practices. All appear to strive to achieve the highest possible 'good' by teaching their followers to believe in a 'Supreme Being' or 'deity', sometimes called God, Allah, Brahman. They accept that 'Being' as all powerful and the creator of the universe.

Every religion has a set of doctrines and codes of behaviour found in a sacred book eg. Bible, Koran, Bhagavad-Gita, and educated ministers eg. priests, rabbis, receive much training to teach these laws and codes and how believers should act and worship their Supreme Being. There is usually some sort of initiation into the religion such as baptism as well as a series of special festivals in the year, eg. Christian Easter, Jewish Passover, Muslim Ramadan. Furthermore, each has its own religious articles such as crucifixes, beads, rosaries, to aid such worship. In addition each religion has beliefs about what happens after death and has certain rituals and customs practised when the person is dying or has died (Neuberger 1987). Nevertheless it must be noted that the degree to which people observe these practices and the strength of these beliefs varies.

In order for nurses to thoughtfully consider other people's spiritual beliefs it is important that they appreciate the basic differences between different sorts of faiths and, indeed, ways of living without a set of religious beliefs ; atheism, agnosticism and secular humanism. Spiritual issues have been defined elsewhere as those that are concerned with personal meaning or how we make sense of the world around us (Burnard 1987). That meaning may be framed in religious terms or it may not. The person who adopts an atheistic, agnostic or secular humanistic position is still creating meaning, it is just that such meaning does not necessarily include a concept of God. It is worth considering, then, the basic tenets of the major religions of the world and the non-religious philosophies that enable people to create meaning.

Whilst Christianity can be divided into at least the Orthodox Church, the Protestant Church and the Roman Catholic Church, there are certain tenets of faith that are common to all three. Within each of the main divisions also exist a wide range of different sects and denominations. All major Christian churches believe in the historical significance of Jesus of Nazareth as the son of God, born of a virgin. The essence of Christianity can be identified in the Apostle's Creed:

> I believe in God the Father Almighty, Creator of heaven and earth: and in Jesus Christ his only Son, our Lord who was conceived by the Holy Spirit, born of the Virgin Mary: suffered under Pontius Pilate, was crucified, dead and buried, he descended into hell; the third day he rose again from the dead and ascended into heaven; is seated at the right hand of God the Father Almighty; from thence he shall come to judge the quick and the dead. I believe in the Holy Ghost; the holy Catholic Church; the Communion of Saints; the Forgiveness of sins; the Resurrection of the body, and the life of the world to come. Amen.

The word 'Catholic' in this passage refers to the notion of universality and is not synonymous with the 'Roman Catholic Church'. Christians of all denominations (and a great many of them are described by Sampson [1982]), celebrate the following principle festivals: Christmas, Lent, Good Friday, Easter Sunday and Whitsun (Pentecost). However, there are a great number of variations of practice in individual denominations and sects. It cannot be assumed that all Christians believe the same things beyond the basic tenets identified above. The theological and doctrinal position adopted by different denominations varies greatly as does the attention paid to the role of ritual and ceremony. These variations are vitally important to individual believers and are well articulated by Sampson (1982) and Rumbold (1986).

Judaism

Judaism is a religion essentially of a particular people, the Jews. The history of Judaism and much more of its theological basis can be found in the Old Testament of the Holy Bible. The Law of the Jewish people is written in the Torah, or first five books of the Old Testament. They await the Messiah and do not recognise Jesus of Nazareth as that Messiah. Important Jewish festivals include: Rosh Hashanah (Jewish New Year), Yom Kippur (the Day of Atonement), Succoth (Feast of Tabernacles), Simchath Torah (Rejoicing in the Law), Chanukah (the Feast of Esther), Purim (the Feast of Lots), Pesach

22

(the Passover) and Tishah B'Av (Mourning for the Destruction of the Temple). Orthodox Jews require their food to be prepared following a specific ritual and abstain from certain types of meat, notably pork.

Hinduism

Hinduism is an ancient religion, originally centred in India and Nepal but which has spread wherever Indians have settled. Hindu's believe that there are many Gods but that all of these are manifestations of one God. Hinduism has no fixed creed and is a very diverse religion. There are a variety of schools of Hindu philosophy and a number of separate religions have developed from it including Buddhism. In the Hindu religion the cow is regarded as a sacred animal and therefore beef is not eaten.

Islam

The religion of Islam is followed by Muslims. Islam, literally, means submission and Muslims are committed to submitting themselves to the will of God. In the Islamic faith, God is called Allah and Muslims believe Him to be the one true God. The Islamic faith calls for its followers to believe absolutely in the will of God and teaches obedience. They consider Mohammed to be the last great prophet following chronologically after the Jewish prophets and Jesus Christ and they follow his teachings. Again, for Muslims animals used for food need to be prepared in a ritual manner.

Clearly, it cannot be claimed that this is an exhaustive description of the religions under discussion nor is it claimed that it is a comprehensive listing of all the world's religions. As we have noted, there is already a considerable literature on the topic, to which the reader is referred. It is important in this context, however, to note the considerable differences between the ways in which different cultures give meaning to religious experience. Given the multi-cultural nature of our society, it is important that all nurses have some appreciation of these varieties of religious interpretation and respect for the differences between them.

Non religious beliefs

Finally, we may consider the issues of atheism and agnosticism. Both are dimensions of spirituality in that both are aspects of some people's belief systems or their attempts to create meaning. Both may be equally respected in the manner that 'religious' beliefs are respected.

Atheism

Atheism is the unequivocal denial of the possible existence of God. The atheist is the 'unbeliever', the person who does not believe in God. It is interesting to ponder on our individual reaction to such a position. For instance, it is possible to respond by seeing such a person as 'wrong', or that such a person needs only to reflect further for clarification or that they need more education in order to bring them to the truth. Or can they be accepted as they are? Various reactions are possible; the least acceptable seems to be the notion that somehow the believer is 'right' and the unbeliever is 'wrong'. Belief in God must necessarily involve a 'leap of faith' (Kierkegaard 1959). There can be no ultimate scientific proof of the existence or non-existence of God. Individuals either believe or do not believe. Neither does the position of unbelief necessarily preclude any sort of moral position. An unbeliever is quite as able to lead a moral life as is a believer. Indeed, Simone de Beauvoir argued that the unbelievers had to lead a 'more moral' life that the believers for, as there was no final arbiter of right and wrong for the unbelievers, they were necessarily thrown back on their own decision making as a guide to conduct. The believer can be 'forgiven': the unbeliever must forgive him/herself.

The atheist has to look beyond a concept of God for meaning. That they have to do that does not mean that they do not have spiritual needs. The spiritual needs of the atheist (in terms of a search for meaning) are just as vital as they are for the believer. Some atheists find that sense of meaning in secular humanism. Secular humanism should not be confused with 'humanistic psychology' (Shaffer 1978). The base argument of secular humanism is best outlined by Blackham (1968). Briefly, the argument is this: persons are alone in that there is no God. Because they are alone, they are responsible for themselves. They also have a joint responsibility for all other persons. In acting for themselves, they should act as though they were acting for all mankind. To do less than this is selfishness and not, so Blackham

24

argues, secular humanism. Such a philosophy offers an immediate sense of meaning: the atheist is responsible for him/herself and for others. As a result, the 'golden rule' applies: 'treat others as we would wish to be treated'. This then, is the basis for morality and for meaning without recourse to belief in God.

Agnosticism

The agnostic, on the other hand, is in a slightly different position. The agnostic argues that, because it is impossible to prove or disprove the existence of God, silence on the issue is the only wise position (Bullock and Stallybrass 1977). The agnostic is neither believer or unbeliever, he holds the view that discussion about the matter is necessarily misplaced, in the end, because such an issue can only ever be a matter of faith. Again, such a position does not, of itself, rule out the need for meaning or morality. The agnostic, like the atheist, still needs to discover or invest life with meaning in what they do or how they live. Some may argue that the only meaning that can be found in life is that which individuals invest in it (Kopp 1972). In other words, there is no ultimate meaning for the way things are: people bring meaning to their actions. Meaning, therefore, is an intrinsic concept and dependent upon the individual's reasoning or perception.

These are two thumbnail sketches of two positions alternative to that of belief in God. There is, of course, another position, that of the person who either does not know whether or not he/she believes is God and a further position, that of the person who does not believe such issues to be important. It is argued here that such positions are just as valid as are those adopted by those who would claim to be believers.

There are many situations in which such positions need to be considered in nursing. As we have seen, one of the questions asked on admission of a patient may relate to that person's 'religion'. Such a question leaves no doubt that the accepted position is that of 'believer'. Indeed, it is quite possible that many patients, in this culture, faced with the question and uncertain about their own beliefs, will answer 'Church of England' or 'Catholic', whether or not they are members of those churches, in order not to embarrass themselves. It may take considerable bravery to answer 'none' or 'atheist' in these circumstances! We need to think long and hard about how we may pose questions of belief or unbelief without making such questions leading questions.

Second, it is necessary to consider the sorts of value-judgements nurses may make about other people's belief systems. If the nurse is a believer, is there a harsh judgement of the unbeliever? If, on the other hand, the nurse is an unbeliever, is the believer dismissed? It is important that there is an acknowledgement that either belief system may not coincide with that of the patient. Nor is it appropriate that nurses proselytise or evangelise for either position. Nurses, in the role of carers, are not required to convert others to belief or unbelief.

There are other, more delicate questions. Acceptance, for instance of the fact that the unbeliever may not see the need for the conventional funeral service. 'secular' forms of service are available through national secular societies. It may also need to be acknowledged that death may not be a fearful event for the unbeliever. Nor need it be a fearful event for unbelieving relatives.

In Marx's vision of an ideal society, religion does not exist. Members of society are fulfilled as human beings, they control their own destinies and work together for the common good. To Marx, religion is an illusion which eases the pain produced by exploitation and oppression (Haralambos 1980). For some, Marxism may become a religion without a God.

Humanistic psychology may serve the same purpose. This is a branch of psychology involving the study of individuals as human beings with their thoughts, feelings and experiences. It is concerned with human growth and individual fulfilment involving both 'determinism', the view that behaviour is determined by various factors outside the person's control, and 'freedom' the view that behaviour is a function of personal choice or free will (Nye 1986).

It could be stated however, that different religious beliefs can also coincide with such ideas on the conduct of life. Myco (1985) notes it would be wrong to suggest a Christian cannot be essentially a Humanist or that a Humanist must be a complete rationalist who denies any supernatural explanation. However it seems that the main criticism against Humanists is that they are too Utopian in believing that it is a good environment and a society which keeps humans happy and will make everyone behave well, knowing it is in their best interest to do so.

Some may argue that individuals must search for and work out their own ultimate solutions and meaning - individuation (Haralambos 1980), whilst others consider the consequences of not believing in a God. According to Myco (1985), self affirmation and self preservation are synonymous in that they both imply the overcoming of something which potentially threatens or denies the self and which may produce anxiety and fear. Philosophers such as Spinoza sought to establish an outlook which could liberate people from oppression of fear. By accepting the concept that there is no life after death, the non believers reduce their anxiety, although they may fear the act of dying, as will all humans.

Spiritual neutrality

The whole of the debate, so far, has focused on people who have spiritual beliefs or on those who look to other belief systems for meaning. What has been left out is any discussion of those who have *no* particular belief systems or faith. It seems likely, too, that there are those for whom consideration of such systems is not particularly important. It is easy, if one is a believer (and whatever the nature of the belief) to imagine that *everyone* is interested, either positively or negatively, in the spiritual domain. It seems possible, however, that there are many for whom the idea of spirituality is not particularly important. Unless we were to argue that the spiritual side of the person is necessarily integral to a notion of what it means to be a person, such an idea is flawed. Everyday life with other people suggests that there is enough anecdotal evidence for the idea of a category of people for whom spiritual ideas play little or no part. The religious person may see such people as ripe for conversion. Possibly the atheist seems him or her in a similar light. Perhaps, though, the 'spiritually neutral' person can take or leave spirituality, atheism and agnosticism. Nor does it seem right to automatically group such people into the category 'agnostic'. The spiritually neutral person does *not* fit into such a category for, as we have seen, to be agnostic is to reject notions of God. The spiritually neutral person finds the concepts of God and of atheism as unnecessary to understanding the world.

Values

Simmons (1982) has compiled a list of one hundred general value statements which are meant to make individuals more aware of what values are and what they mean to each particular person, eg. having good health; having a close relationship; fighting to preserve the natural world. But Simon and Clark, cited by Tschudin (1986), suggest that for individuals to really own a value, they not only need the freedom to acquire it and choose from alternatives, but they also need to prize it and cherish it and be willing to make it known to others. Individuals then need to act on it and behave in such a way as to show that they have made a choice.

Frankl (1964) argues that people find meaning through values. Creative values, those discovered through what is done, particularly through helping others; experiential values, discovered through appreciation of people and events; attitudinal values discovered through reacting to unfortunate circumstances over which there is no control, such as other people's suffering.

Yet values appear less fixed and more dynamic than beliefs. As Tschudin (1986) notes, when young, things are often seen in terms of black and white. But experiences of life and mixing with others, shape and change the values people hold. The process of choosing, prizing and acting on, is therefore a constantly changing one. For some people, more and more things have values; yet for others, as they grow older, fewer and fewer values emerge.

Values clarification

One approach to coming to terms with meaning is through the process known as values clarification. A values clarification questionnaire is included as appendix III of this book for use with students. If we are clear about what we value and feel to be important, we can more easily cope with many of the dilemmas that face us both in our personal and professional lives. Such clarification can arise out of discussion and dispute with friends and colleagues. It can also be aided by conscious consideration of a number of difficult ethical issues and matters of principle. If we can be clear about what it is that we believe and why we hold those beliefs, we may be less tempted to ignore or dispute the belief and value systems of others. Arguably, the health professions are not the place for evangelising or proselytising for a particular set of values or beliefs. We need to be both aware of our own beliefs and values and accepting of those of others.

Berne (1972) suggested that people tend to adopt certain life positions in relation to others. In this simple, economical way of considering life values and attitudes towards others, Berne suggests four possible life positions:

- I'm OK - You're OK
- I'm OK - You're not OK
- I'm not OK - You're not OK
- I'm not OK - You're OK

The person who develops the 'I'm OK - You're OK' position is essentially positive about themselves and about others. In being clear about their own values and themselves, they are able to accept the values and differences of other people. They are positive about themselves and about others.

The person who adopts the 'I'm OK - You're not OK ' positions is positive about their own values but are highly critical of others. Sometimes this is because they distrust or are uncertain of their own values. Sometimes it is because they hold their values so dogmatically that they find it impossible to believe that other sorts of values can be held. Such people can appear arrogant and distant in their relationships with others.

The person who adopts the 'I'm not OK - You're not OK' position doubts both his own values and those of others. Essentially, he takes a fairly dim view of both himself and other people. This negative view of life tends to be self-reinforcing. The more this person looks for weaknesses in himself and other people in general, the more he finds those weaknesses to be evident! For this person, relationships are doomed to failure because of the inherent weaknesses in all people.

Almost as distressing as the above life position is that of the person who adopts the I'm not OK - You're OK position. This person feels that the rest of the world is superior. Everyone else manages and copes whilst he battles and yet fails.

The process of clarifying values can help to establish or reestablish the position of 'I'm OK - You're OK. In the end, this position must be the best one for the health professional to adopt both personally and professionally. The other life positions either tend to lead towards very painful lives or they cause the health professional to develop a bitter and cynical view of their jobs and of their clients.

Berne's analysis of life positions is also a useful framework through which to consider how clients view their lives. Very often, the person who seeks out a health professional for help with problems in living or emotional difficulties is adopting the 'You're OK - I'm not OK' position in relation to that health professional. They have often adopted that position in relation to other people in their lives as well. Just acknowledging the style of life position that is being played out in the client-professional relationship can help in attempting to redress the balance. Berne's analysis offers a simple yet effective way of exploring relationships.

Meditation

Another approach to the question of meaning is through contemplation and thoughtfulness, via meditation. Clearly, all sorts of other approaches are possible, from pastoral counselling, through intensive psychotherapy to help from Church workers. Discussion with friends is another approach to tackling these fundamental questions of meaning. It is also important to differentiate questions of meaning from clinical depression. The depressed person, after all, may exhibit some or all of the above characteristics. When clinical depression exists, it should be treated through one of the many psychological and pharmacological approaches available. Why, then, the recommendation of meditation?

In the end, questions of meaning involve what Kierkegaard called a 'leap of faith'. It seems unlikely that there will ever be factual, empirical evidence to help us to untangle questions of meaning. In the end, we have to decide for ourselves. What we believe, what sustains us, can only come through inner conviction. That inner conviction cannot be given to us by another person, we can only experience it (or not experience it) for ourselves. In the normal flow of life we are constantly being caught up in the processes of thinking about our work, our families, our commitments and so on. We rarely have time to sit and quietly think through our beliefs or lack of them. If nothing else, meditation can offer a time of peace and quiet during or after which we may be able to apply ourselves to thinking about our own beliefs and meaning systems.

Faith

Faith is a word that is used to refer to a belief or assent to something that cannot be seen, so allowing an individual to believe in a 'Higher Being' that cannot be directly seen or heard. Burrell and Wright (1983) recognise this is widely discussed in the theological literature.

Carson (1989b) considers faith has a developmental quality. It matures and changes in response to life events and has been discussed by the theorists, Fowler, Aden, Westerhoff and Erikson, all of whom from their various research, have evolved discrete stages of faith. According to Fowler cited by Carson (1989b), it is faith that acknowledges life as meaningful and gives individuals meaning and purpose in life. Whilst it can be religious, it can be centred on a career, country, family, money or even self.

Hope

Stoll (1979) states that hope is to have a future, a sense of the possible, without which a person is left with despair. Others have documented situations where the presence or lack of hope has meant the difference between survival or death (Frankl 1964) and Weisman (1979) identifies hope as a prerequisite for effective coping with the demands and challenges of such illnesses as cancer. It could be said therefore, that hope strengthens individuals to deal with the situations and stresses that accompany life (Travelbee 1971).

Carson (1989b) reviews the multidisciplinary writings of philosophers, theologians and nurses and reveals that there are four major themes that are associated with hope. The first two are, orientation towards the future and the setting of goals. Individuals must be able to imagine a future outcome or have a goal in order to hope. The next is acting to meet those goals. With hope individuals seem to act, move and achieve. Without hope, they are often dull and listless and moribund. Finally there is establishing interpersonal relationships. For this there is trust. Trust in others, oneself and in the environment around.

Summary

Religious and non religious belief systems have been reviewed. A brief overview of values has also been given. All would appear to give individuals some kind of meaning and purpose to their lives. In addition it seems that both faith and hope are an integral part of spirituality. However whatever religion, non religion, values, faith and hope individuals adopt, it would seem that facing life without some kind of ideological framework could lead to a certain degree of uncertainty and possible distress particularly in times of traumatic life experiences.

32

3 Spirituality and nursing practice

The concept of spirituality appears to be an important aspect of nursing practice. This section will therefore examine this relationship by firstly outlining its relevance/importance to nursing. This will then be followed by a critical review of the nursing research in order to establish to what extent patients' spiritual needs are met. Possible reasons for the inadequate consideration of such issues will be discussed. Spiritual aspects of acute illness will then be highlighted.

Relevance/importance

The principle codes governing nursing practice acknowledge nurses' responsibility to respect patients' values and beliefs (International Council Nurses - I.C.N 1973, United Kingdom Central Council UKCC 1984). The UKCC's recently revised Code of Conduct (UKCC 1992) also asks practitioners to recognise and respect the uniqueness and dignity of patients/clients. This could be seen as merely requiring nurses to passively avoid offending their patients. From earlier discussion, it could be argued that spirituality is possibly the deepest requirement of the self, which if met, makes it possible for people to function with meaningful identity and purpose - a sense of wholeness. Ensuring spiritual safety and well being therefore demands active consideration and to ignore this would be a gross omission. This is all the more relevant in today's British multicultural society where care is provided for people of different ethnic and religious backgrounds by caregivers with divergent religious beliefs and spiritual inclinations.

Society generally now appears to have a heightened sense of its own mortality and interest in the search for meaning (Inglehart 1983, Garcia and Maitland 1983, Kapleau 1989, King 1989). In recent years there have been a series of major natural disasters around the world. For example, earthquakes and mudslides, with the loss of thousands of lives; the sudden violent deaths of the football supporters at Hillsborough; and the victims of the Zebrugge ferry disaster. Ley and Corless (1988) argue that the mythic 'sense of control' has now been shaken and this has added impetus to the movement to turn away from the reliance on science and technology and turn instead to the search for meaning.

Burnard (1987) notes that the range of experiences of spiritual problems is wide and may be met by nurses in a variety of settings. Since the early 1980's when the changing pattern of health needs became widely recognised (Cox 1982), the number of the elderly in the population has increased and Brooke (1987) and Forbis (1988) discuss the importance of spiritual well being for this age group. They point out that as people age, the need for inner serenity becomes important and spiritual beliefs can offer a means for reconciliation and an understanding of life. It is often the spiritual dimension that provides meaning to age related experiences and enables the elderly to cope with the problems that result from illness and old age. Erikson, cited by Forbis (1988), in his developmental staging for the elderly adult, states that people must resolve a conflict between spiritual integrity and despair before achieving life satisfaction in later life. Because spirituality can help people transcend the physical, nurses' support in helping the elderly fulfil their spiritual needs may help them meet their developmental needs, as well as resulting in greater life satisfaction.

Henderson (1989) considers that the AIDS crisis has given a new priority to therapeutic measures for people facing a chronic or terminal disease. As Burkhardt and Nagai-Jacobson (1985), and Carson et al (1990) note, faced with the reality of physical death and losses involved, patients may question the meaning of their lives, changes in significant relationships and raise other spiritual issues. It would seem that attending to these spiritual needs is essential in order to alleviate suffering and restore well being.

Meeting patients' spiritual needs

Although the importance of meeting patients' spiritual needs has gained emphasis (Granstrom 1985, Soeken and Carson 1987, Carson 1989a), it has been noted that nurses have limited awareness of patients' spiritual needs and some American studies identify little evidence that they actually provide spiritual care (Highfield and Cason 1983, Soeken and Carson 1986).

Other American nursing writers do appear to cover various aspects of spirituality and nursing practice (Frye and Long 1985, Burkhardt and Nagai-Jacobson 1985, Bowers 1987, Peterson and Nelson 1987). However much of this is based on personal experience and no empirical evidence. Such topics are not totally neglected by the British nursing literature (Sampson 1982, McGilloway and Myco 1985, Burnard 1986, 1987, 1988 a,b,c, Neuberger 1987, Green 1989 a,b,c, Morrison 1990) but many are limited to religious practices, particularly those surrounding death.

There also appears little empirical evidence about how patients cope spiritually with illness and it would seem without this knowledge it is difficult for nurses to consider appropriate spiritual care to meet their specific spiritual needs. Nevertheless an English study by Simsen (1986) using triangulation, revealed patients had a constant need to make sense of their circumstances, to find meaning in the events of their day, their relationships, their life.

The sample study was small - 45 interviews but a number of set criteria ensured the inclusion of people with a variety of beliefs. However because of the small sample number the results cannot be generalised. Nevertheless the study showed there was a willingness by these patients to talk about their beliefs and it appeared personal beliefs and practices rated more highly than institutionalised forms. The habit of passing all matters spiritual and religious to the chaplain may not be appropriate for all patients.

There has been other research investigating patients' spirituality (Miller 1985, Reed 1987, Sodestrom and Martinson 1987). Although they are comparatively small American studies and because of cultural and health care system differences, the results cannot be generalised, they are worth noting.

Miller (1985) examined the relationship of loneliness, spiritual well being and chronic illness. Reporting on a sample of 64 adults with rheumatoid arthritis and 64 healthy adults, the chronically ill group had significantly higher levels of spiritual well being when compared to the healthy group.

Reed (1987) also discovered that a group of terminally ill hospitalised adult patients exhibited a greater spiritual perspective than the non hospitalised and non terminally ill hospitalised adult groups.

Both these findings raise questions regarding the role of spirituality as an enhancement to coping in the face of either a chronic or terminal illness. Furthermore, Sodestrom and Martinson (1987) found that oncology nurses needed to recognise the importance of assessing cancer patients' reliance on religious faith and subsequent use of spiritual coping strategies.

It may be that through further research about patients' spirituality in this country, there could be a greater understanding of patients' coping strategies and nurses could help patients manage illness more effectively.

Therefore whilst it appears spirituality is not neglected by the nursing literature more research evidence is required to identify patients' spiritual needs related to illness and in addition, more evidence is required to highlight the extent of nurses' awareness of their patients' resources and coping strategies. Without this it is difficult to judge to what extent patients' spiritual needs are met although it does suggest that the concept of spirituality is not addressed as effectively as it should be.

Reasons for inadequate consideration of spiritual issues

The reasons why there appears to be no united effort made to ensure spiritual needs are met consistently can be identified by examining some of the problems inherent in addressing spirituality and nursing practice.

One problem noted by McCavery (1985) is that spiritual assessment and care are subjective and their success rests upon the meaning of conversations between individual nurses and patients and the degree of trust and understanding within such relationships. Furthermore the role of the nurse in relation to the role of the chaplain is as yet ill defined (Ley and Corless 1988).

Ellis (1980) suggests that as nursing has become so biologically oriented, spiritual matters are a source of discomfort and embarrassment for the nurses. Granstrom (1985) states that fear may be a reason for nurses' reluctance to incorporate spiritual care into nursing practice, fear of getting into a situation they cannot handle, fear of intruding on a patient's privacy and fear of being converted or confused in their own belief system. Morrison (1990) believes that nurses generally find spiritual health care hard to articulate because it raises so may questions about life in which there are no specific answers or provable certainties. To make any statements in such an area is to make oneself extremely vulnerable. It is easier for nurses to remain quiet and get on with things in their own way without too much scrutiny of their own beliefs or those of others.

Granstrom (1985) argues that whilst pluralism is a tremendous strength of a society that allows for religious, political and individual freedom, it means that nurses and patients may also embrace a variety of ideologies and philosophies which may or may not be conflicting. As a result much of the literature concerning spiritual care has been directed at a particular religion or denominational belief system. Whilst being helpful, this may have resulted in confusing nurses as to how to give spiritual care to patients who do not embrace these particular beliefs.

In addition, nurses appear to vary greatly in spiritual awareness and Fish and Shelly cited by Soeken and Carson (1986) suggest it is because of the inadequacy of nurses' own spiritual resources or spiritual well being that there is a lack of consideration about such issues. Soeken and Carson (1986) investigated this by examining the relationship between the spiritual well being of nurses and their attitudes towards providing spiritual care for patients. Although a positive correlation was demonstrated between the spiritual well being of nurses and their perceptions of the health professional's role in spiritual care, Soeken and Carson (1986) note that this does not necessarily mean that these nurses actually incorporated spiritual interventions into their nursing care. A positive attitude does not guarantee action. However unless nurses address their own values and belief systems and what gives their life meaning and purpose, they are likely to be uncomfortable in dealing with patients' spiritual quest (Granstrom 1985).

Spiritual aspects of acute illness

For the purpose of this study, acute illness refers to those patients who are admitted to Intensive Care/Coronary care units in a critical medical state of ill health. They often face imminent death and this can possibly be avoided by intensive or high dependency nursing. Such patients would include those who had suffered myocardial infarctions.

Society's advancement in technology and rapid advance in medical science, has resulted in improved health status and marked increase in life expectancy and so altered the nature of nursing (Cluff 1986). As machines have taken over many of the tasks nurses once performed, so has the emphasis on the technological aspects of care increased, sometimes shadowing the concern for spiritual and humanitarian needs. As McCavery (1985) notes it has been easy, particularly in high technology acute areas, to forget that caring is the concern for the totality of the recipient of nursing - the physical, emotional, social and spiritual dimensions of that person.

Yet the crisis of critical illness may present for patients and their relatives, the initial encounter with the spiritual self and the first examination of the meaning and purpose in life (Shaffer 1991). Whilst it is difficult to ascertain the feelings of individuals when they find themselves in a life threatening situation (since individuals respond in different ways), the need for meaning is rarely stronger than when acutely ill patients witness the death of others or anticipate their own (McCavery 1985). Autton (1980) claims that illness and the threat of death forces individuals to make sense of their experiences in the world. Until these experiences are put into some kind of framework of meaning, restlessness, uneasiness, anxiety, doubt and bitterness hamper the recovery to health.

Whilst pain is a subjective phenomenon, patients often feel powerless and controlled by the amount and quality of pain (McCaffery 1983). This is true of the intense chest pain associated with myocardial infarction. Patients may experience a certain vulnerability and dependency as the relief of the symptoms depend on the standards of care administered by the nursing staff. In a somewhat mechanistic environment, suffering pain and facing the possibility of death, the need to receive love is intensified (McCavery 1985).

Where patients no longer feel able to affect their own personal destinies but are controlled by the disease process, there is a feeling of powerlessness. This in turn may leave them feeling 'naked and buffeted' by the illness (Soeken and Carson 1987). If spiritual well being is an empowering state where life has meaning, it could be said that when the sense of power has gone, so too has the sense of spiritual well being.

Furthermore, it is likely that the individuals who lose this control of their bodies feel that they are no longer worthy as useful, independent and dignified humans. Feeling different from and inferior to others can lead to the desire to retreat from all interactions. Isolation can be so complete that they sink lower into feelings of worthlessness, utter loneliness and spiritual deprivation.

Ashworth (1990) notes that it is intensive care nurses who seek to provide this much needed support to all in the middle of this emotionally charged atmosphere, so attempting to restore spiritual well being. But Fromant (1988) suggests that even these nurses have faced feelings of inadequacy and distress and isolation when caring for their patients. Continuous close contact with distressed and frightened families can also subject nurses to their own spiritual distress. Unless nurses are aware of this and develop their own coping strategies, they may become less able to give spiritual support.

Summary

It has been argued that spirituality is an important concept related to nursing practice and in reviewing the literature, it appears more research is necessary to judge the extent to which patients' spiritual needs are met.

It is suggested that nurses inadequately consider spiritual issues and various reasons for this have been put forward. It may be that if nurses' knowledge and understanding about spirituality were improved, then the spiritual dimension of patients' could be addressed more effectively.

Furthermore, in highlighting the spiritual aspects of acute illness, there is recognition of the spiritual dimension of nurses. Without consideration of the spiritual nature of nurses and the impact on patients, the subject of spirituality and nursing practice is one sided and incomplete.

4 Spirituality and the nursing process

Since it has been argued that spirituality is an important concept related to nursing practice, consideration is necessary as to how it can be incorporated into patient care. A holistic and planned systematic approach to care may facilitate this: holistic, involving all elements of the person as already discussed and a planned systematic approach, involving four phases, assessment, planning, implementation and evaluation - the nursing process (Yura and Walsh 1983). This chapter will consider spiritual assessment and providing spiritual care.

Spiritual assessment

It would seem that if spiritual needs are to be met then nurses must not only have some awareness of the importance of patients' spiritual needs but also include some sort of spiritual assessment in the initial assessment, in order to accurately identify specific spiritual needs.

However Clifford and Gruca (1987) and Carson (1989c) consider that this is often a neglected area. The patients' religious affiliations may be the only portion of the assessment data related to spiritual aspects and as Burnard

(1988b) points out, many unbelievers (or those who have not considered such issues) nervous of expressing such a position may find it more 'comfortable' to have themselves marked down as 'Church of England' or 'other religion'. It appears further research should examine this suspected lack of consideration of spiritual assessment. This issue was discussed in more detail in the previous chapter.

A number of different approaches to spiritual assessment have been identified. Some authors have developed specific spiritual history guides which may be used to identify specific areas of concern (Stoll 1979, O'Brien 1982). They certainly appear to provide an in-depth analysis of spiritual needs and address more than religious affiliations but they would seem to be time consuming to complete. Other authors suggest more general questions during the initial assessment concerning such topics as religion, meaning and hope (Shelly 1982, Byrne 1985, Peterson and Nelson 1987, Ferszt and Taylor 1988).

However these guidelines were developed in America where attitudes towards discussing such intimate and personal details are possibly more open. Further refinement of such tools and the development of new measures suitable for use in Britain may enable expansion of the understanding of this under researched area.

Nevertheless, Peterson and Nelson (1987) suggest that assessment of patients' spiritual component requires more than questioning. By observing the patients and their environment (whether they have religious objects with them, whether they perform rituals/practices), their behaviour with family and friends and their facial expressions indicating fear, doubt, depression or despair, the nurses can obtain valuable information.

Carson (1989c) provides a detailed list of observations to be made in a spiritual assessment and this, with Stoll's (1979) questions relating to four areas of concern, the concept of God or deity, sources of hope and strength, the significance of religious practices and rituals and the relationship between spiritual beliefs and state of health, appears to provide a comprehensive format for assessment which could perhaps be adapted for use in Britain (Figure 4.1).

Concept of God	1. Is religion or God important to you? If so, can you describe how? 2. Do you use prayer in your life? If so, does prayer benefit you in any way? 3. Do you believe God or a deity is involved in your personal life? If so, how? 4. What is your God or deity like?
Sources of strength and hope	1. Who are your support people? 2. Who is the most important person in your life? 3. Are people available to you when you are in need? 4. Who or what provides you with strength and hope?
Religious practices	1. Is your religious faith helpful to you? 2. Are there any religious practices that are meaningful to you? 3. Has your illness affected your religious practices? 4. Are there any religious books or symbols that are helpful to you?

Figure 4.1 Areas to be covered in a spirituality interview (adapted from Stoll in Carson 1989c, p.159)

However Shelly (1982) discusses the importance of listening for clues. She suggests patients make references to spiritual concerns more often than nurses actually hear them. It may be that the best approach to spiritual assessment avoids asking one question after another. Instead the questions could be used to respond to non verbal, as well as verbal clues that indicate the presence of a spiritual need. Furthermore as Carson (1989c) notes, it is important for nurses undertaking such an assessment, to approach the patients with acceptance and sensitivity and build up a trusting empathetic relationship.

Providing spiritual care

O'Brien (1982) notes that any nursing intervention for patients includes those actions which indicate caring. O'Brien (1982) describes caring as:

> ... indicating to the person that he/she is important or significant and is worth someone taking the trouble to be concerned about" (O'Brien 1982).

Whilst it appears care and caring are complex concepts, they are frequently seen as ordinary, simple and easy to put into practice (Pearson 1991). Yet caring involves being assertive, giving support, providing assistance in growing and fostering empowerment (not control). It involves an attitude of helping, sharing, nurturing and loving (O'Brien 1982).

Certain writings on the provision of spiritual care direct attention to specialised groups; oncology patients (Granstrom 1985) hospice services (Ley and Corless 1988), patients with critical illnesses (Shelly 1982), patients with AIDS (Belcher et al 1989), the elderly (Cluff 1986) and patients in the rehabilitation setting (Bowers 1987). It would seem spiritual care can be applied to any and all of these areas. Yet there remains little evidence to support what constitutes effective spiritual care per se and how it differs from the general concept of care.

O'Brien (1982) suggests that spiritual care, as the concept of care itself, is very broad and may encompass many types of nursing behaviour. It may involve more specifically the unique relationship and rapport between nurses and patients, where nurses must respect and understand their patients' values and beliefs, be they religious or non-religious, even though they may differ from their own. They must offer love, kindness, mercy and understanding and such qualities which add meaning to life and can bring increased solace and comfort.

Some writers recognise that one of the most essential nursing interventions during spiritual distress is 'presence' (Carson 1989c, Shaffer 1991). That is 'being there' in the physical sense and 'being with' in the psychological sense. This type of intervention corresponds to what Travelbee (1971) refers to as 'the therapeutic use of self' and which is discussed by Ersser (1991). This is enhanced by empathetic listening implying genuineness, trust and positive regard, which is reflected in the interpersonal rapport between the patients and nurses. In addition, therapeutic touch may for some provide emotional comfort and support during spiritual distress (Shaffer 1991).

However, determining the appropriateness of therapeutic touch requires nurses to be sensitive as to how patients might respond to a comforting hand.

It seems that many writers regard listening as an essential aspect of spiritual care (O'Brien 1982, Peterson 1985, Carson 1989c). This is also an important element of counselling. Burnard (1987) who advocates a non-directive client centred approach to counselling as described by Rogers (1967) also highlights the importance of such skills as listening, questioning and empathy when dealing with such patients. However he also notes that for the spiritually distressed, basic counselling skills are not enough. For some patients, nurses as counsellors may need to deal with the release of emotions or the quiet talking through thoughts and feelings or long periods of silences but always with the acknowledgement of their patients' feelings of meaninglessness and lack of purpose in life.

Underpinning the approaches to helping patients with their spirituality, is the need for nurses to clarify their own values and beliefs. It may be extremely difficult to counsel others in this area of spirituality if nurses are unclear of their own position in relation to beliefs and values. The reason for this is not for the purpose of converting the patients to a particular religious or secular position but to help nurses differentiate between the patients' problems and their own (Labun 1988).

Furthermore, nurses providing spiritual care need to acknowledge that they have limitations and involve others when they do not feel comfortable in dealing with the situation or when the patients want someone else. This may be the chaplain, local clergy or religious advisor (Peterson 1985). Carson (1989c) considers that when nurses are able to approach patients, expecting to learn from them and recognising that they do not have all the answers, they have acquired humility. It is humility that allows nurses to accept both themselves and patients as they are.

Summary

It appears that spiritual assessment is often a neglected aspect of care. Yet without it, it is doubtful that specific spiritual needs/problems can be accurately identified.

The literature offers a number of different approaches to this assessment that includes the important communication skills of questioning, listening and observing. However it would seem that more discussion and research needs to be given to this aspect of care, in order to realistically incorporate this assessment into nursing practice in Britain.

Spiritual care has been discussed and seems to include a variety of nursing interventions eg. the use of 'presence', developing a rapport with patients, counselling skills. Many of these involve those interventions that indicate 'caring'. Indeed many nurses may provide this type of care unconsciously, although spiritual care would also appear to acknowledge patients' feelings of meaninglessness and lack of purpose in life.

It is suggested that spiritual care is therefore not anything that is completely alien to nurses and should not be feared or considered as a 'nice extra'. It is argued that it is in fact a vital ingredient in health care and an essential part of the nurse's role.

5 The study

Spirituality appears a complex, yet significant aspect of nursing. The aim of this study was to explore trained nurses' perceptions of the concept of spirituality both personally and professionally, in order to highlight their knowledge and understanding.

This approach therefore allowed consideration as to how nurses could be assisted to meet the spiritual needs of patients. Furthermore it was hoped that some kind of theoretical and practical model for practice could be put forward for further development.

Quantitative and qualitative research methods

In the nursing literature over the past two-three decades there appears to have been a vast increase in nursing research and theory development. Duffy (1985) argues that in this age of technology and objectivism, quantification of data has been seen as the truly scientific methodology. Meanwhile qualitative research has been of secondary significance, reserved for exploratory studies designed as the preliminary stage of quantitative research.

However, there has been a growing realisation among nurse researchers that quantitative methodologies do not answer all the questions (Treece and Treece 1986). In addition, the value and worth of qualitative data are being recognised by many (Field and Morse 1985, Leininger 1985, Parse et al 1985, Munhall and Oiler 1986, Morse 1991a).

Duffy (1985) offers a comprehensive comparison of the two approaches and the merits and appropriateness of each for nursing research. She notes that their differences are not only concerned with methodology but with philosophy. Quantitative methods attempt to measure phenomena in the form of numbers and are concerned solely with observations of phenomena, where the observers are totally separate and distinct from that which is being studied (Brink and Wood 1989).

In contrast, qualitative methodologies are concerned with understanding the meaning of phenomena, not a readily observable process (Schwartz and Jacobs cited by Duffy 1985). Thus as Brink and Wood (1989) note, qualitative data collection methods are flexible and somewhat unstructured producing data that does not usually take on a numerical form but gives verbatim reports on observable characteristics. They are concerned with 'rich' and 'deep' and 'soft' data (Field and Morse 1985).

Yet a more fundamental difference is one of philosophy. Bryman (1988) states that researchers using quantitative methods take the stance of "determinism" ie. everywhere in the world is subject of causal laws. The way to explain the world scientifically is to collect, measure and count things as they happen in order to test theories and laws. Arising from the branch of philosophy known as logical positivism (Carter 1991), this would seem to be an important dimension to quantitative approaches. This positivist approach is therefore concerned with a deductive process of knowledge attainment, seeking to verify facts and causal relationships in existing theory. Quantitative approaches therefore approach problems from the top down (from theory to practice). Certainly they do seem to offer a systematic, reliable way of classifying and quantifying the world as accurately as possible (Abraham et al 1989).

Nevertheless, Bryman (1988) points out that researchers using qualitative methods appear to consider that perceptions of what is happening in the world are affected by many variables, eg. culture, past experiences, belief systems. Therefore the philosophical dimension to these qualitative approaches is that it is not possible to view the world 'as it is' but only 'as it is believed to be'. Thus qualitative research methodologies involve inductive processes, generating theory from facts obtained within the natural setting of the

47

phenomena (Field and Morse 1985). Hutchinson (1986) refers to this as a bottom up approach to a problem (from practice to theory).

There appears to be several qualitative approaches to studying and discovering how people know and understand their world and include ethnography, phenomenology and grounded theory. Whereas ethnography is grounded in the culture concept and seeks to understand the 'natives' view of a cultural system (Aamodt 1991), phenomenology is used to discover and understand the meaning of human life experiences through analysis of the subjects' descriptions of situations (Leininger 1987). On the other hand, according to Stern (1985), grounded theory is a research method used for searching or relating factors to the research problem in question. The data generated is therefore grounded in fact and from the data, theory evolves.

Thus it appears that researchers using these qualitative methods reject the assumptions of positivism and attempt to humanise the research process. There is an entwining of the observer and phenomena and increased validity, ie. the extent to which the research findings represent reality (Duffy 1985).

It seems therefore, that quantitative methods offer an accurate, systematic way of classifying the world and qualitative methods offer ways of studying people's experiences, beliefs and meanings about life.

The research approach

Because of the nature of the aim of this study, a descriptive qualitative approach, using in depth interviews and modified aspects of grounded theory, appeared the most suitable for this particular project. Exploring people's perceptions about spirituality necessitated an approach that would search out detailed, possibly ambiguous in depth accounts and beliefs about spirituality, so generating rich, soft qualitative data. This corresponded well to the assumptions and philosophical beliefs that characterised the qualitative approaches, as set out by Leininger (1987).

As already stated, grounded theory is one approach to the development of inductive theory and has been described by Glaser and Strauss (1967). It focuses primarily on obtaining people's view points, values and life styles and it also seeks to discover attributes, meanings and characteristics of phenomena.

However the grounded theory method of research goes beyond describing a phenomena, to conceptualising it (Munhall 1989). Stern cited by Munhall (1989) states that:

Grounded theory aims to generate theoretical constructs which explain action in the social context under study (Stern cited by Munhall 1989).

As Hutchinson (1986) explains, grounded theory contains an inherent safeguard against the danger of leaning too heavily on inherited theories. That is, its explanation of key 'social structures or processes' is derived from or grounded in, the empirical data itself.

Furthermore, the generation of grounded theory appears to rely on the inquiring, analytical minds of its researchers. It utilises an inductive approach (from the ground up), using everyday behaviours or organisational patterns to generate theory. Thus the resulting theory not only emerges as an entirely new way of understanding the phenomena from which it is generated, but is inherently relevant to the world from which is emerges (Hutchinson 1986).

For these reasons grounded theory appeared to be of value when addressing this particular research question and related to many of the beliefs and ideas of the researchers.

Nevertheless, criticisms of grounded theory must be noted. Whilst Glaser and Strauss (1967) have described grounded theory, Stern (1985) notes that researchers using this method have encountered a number of problems. Since Glaser and Strauss, both sociologists, described the method in language difficult to understand, this has given rise to a number of different interpretations of the method, which bear only a slight resemblance to the original work. Furthermore some nurse 'scientists', more accustomed to a step by step linear approach, consider that grounded theory, because of its lack of clarity and different approach, is consequently unscientific and unsound.

It could be argued that whilst this research approach is able to prescribe how to do certain sorts of research, it has not yet been fully explored. Furthermore it is open to question as to whether or not it is possible to do 'pure' grounded theory, as is the degree to which grounded theory can be completely differentiated from other sorts of phenomenological and qualitative approaches. Yet if the grounded theory approach cannot be clearly defined and descriptions about how it can be operationalised cannot be given, it may not be possible to defend it as a research approach. It was in the light of these criticisms that modified aspects of grounded theory were used in this study.

The sample

Since the purpose of any qualitative research is to discover meaning and not to measure the distribution of attributes within the population, the question of generalisability is not pertinent. Therefore, as Field and Morse (1985) note, in contrast to quantitative research, the number of subjects in a qualitative study is necessarily small and a random sample is not selected.

For these reasons and because of time constraints, it was decided to interview a small group of approximately 10-15. The aim of this study was to study the perceptions of a group of trained nurses. It therefore seemed appropriate to select participants that were practising qualified nurses. This is known as purposeful sampling. Advocated by Field and Morse (1985), McNeil (1990) and Morse (1991b) as one of several types of sampling in qualitative research, selection of participants occurs according to the needs of the study. In grounded theory this is also known as theoretical sampling (Wilson 1989).

However in the researcher's opinion, the complex nature of the concept of spirituality and type of intimate questions that were going to be posed, demanded other criteria for inclusion. The researcher felt it was important to include those with whom she had an established relationship of trust and who, in her opinion, would be able to openly and clearly articulate their thoughts and feelings. Respondents selected according to the quality of their relationship with the researcher and their ability to articulate and provide explanations for the researcher is known as opportunistic sampling (Agar cited by Field and Morse 1985). Thus two approaches to selecting the respondents were used, purposeful sampling and opportunistic sampling.

Following the suggestions of Morse (1991b), the appropriateness and adequacy of the sample were ensured. The appropriateness of the sample was evaluated throughout the data collection period by examining and reviewing the methods of sampling and determining if the methods used and the sample obtained, facilitated understanding of the research problem, in this case the perceptions of spirituality.

In order to ensure adequacy, that is:

... the sufficiency and quality of data obtained (Morse 1991b).

the amount of information obtained and its relevance and completeness were assessed. After the ninth interview, the researcher became conscious of feeling 'somewhat bored' and of not listening to anything new. Morse (1991b) refers to this stage of data collection as 'saturation'. Therefore it was decided to finish the data collection after the tenth interview since no new aspects/categories were emerging and a great deal of information had already been collected. This closure of the data collection was therefore determined by the amount and quality of data and not by a pre-determined sample size that usually occurs with statistical sampling (Wilson 1989).

Data collection

Interviews were chosen as the method of exploring perceptions of spirituality. Ten trained nurses were interviewed separately using a semi-structured interview schedule. Interviews were tape recorded and then transcribed. On each occasion the respondent's permission was sought. No one refused.

By having just a list of issues and some open questions that had to be covered in each interview, eg. definitions, relevance to nursing practice, the interview was more like a conversation. Topics were discussed as they arose rather than in the order and format prescribed on a questionnaire or in a more structured interview. Open questions were used to elicit this information. The benefits of using such a method of data collection has been noted by Couchman and Dawson (1990). The information gathered in this way is much 'richer' than data collected in a more structured approach.

In order to construct the semi-structured interview schedule, the issues to be covered needed to be clearly identified. Ideas for such issues were generated from the researcher's own experience, Stoll's (1979) spiritual assessment guide and Jacik's (1989) personal spiritual survey. These issues were then put forward to two people who were not in any way involved in the study. This proved helpful since independently they felt that to consider such intimate personal thoughts required time and some consideration. As a result it was decided to ask each respondent, prior to the interview, to spend some time considering spirituality, so that they did not arrive at the interview 'cold'. Each respondent was asked not to discuss his/her thoughts with anyone else, to ensure the perceptions were 'individual'.

The researcher was also concerned about conducting such interviews, probing so deeply into people's personal domain. Questions relating to personal aspects of spirituality were therefore asked during the latter part of the interview, so giving time for the respondents to relax into the situation. Once the interview schedule had been formulated, it was piloted on a person who was not a nurse but who worked in a health care setting where the concept of spirituality was an important part of the philosophy of care.

One of the problems of piloting an interview schedule using a semi-structured approach is that it can never be an exact trial run for subsequent interviews, since a list of questions is not used. However piloting such an interview and its transcription did allow for ambiguities in questioning to be highlighted and corrected, and any tendency to lead the interview, to be modified. In addition, it highlighted the balance in the amount said by the interviewer and the respondent. Furthermore, this pilot interview helped the researcher overcome her anxieties in posing such searching questions and in using a tape recorder to its best advantage. Field and Morse (1985) refer to these anxieties as 'stage fright'.

Although the pilot interview was not intended for use in the main study, the material was extremely valuable. Rowan (1981) recognises that much can be learnt from pilot work if it is well described. So with the pilot interviewee's permission, the interview has been included as a case study.

Each interview took approximately 30-45 minutes, during which certain techniques were used to encourage the respondents eg. using silences, acknowledging with 'hm' and 'yes', so giving permission for the respondents to continue. According to Field and Morse (1985) these are some of the best ways of increasing the richness and depth of the data. However the researcher was also very aware of the danger of moving the respondent along too quickly. So techniques that 'reflected' and 'summarised' what had been said, were used eg. "It seems to me that ...", "Am I correct in saying that ...". In using this approach, an attempt was therefore made to enter the perceptual world of the other person without influencing or leading them. This seemed consistent with the grounded theory approach to research (Hutchinson 1986).

The researcher was also aware of the ease with which this type of research could turn into a counselling session and was anxious that this should not occur. One of the aims of both counselling and this type of research is to explore the perceptual world of the other person. Whilst in counselling the result should be a therapeutic interaction (Burnard 1989), as already shown, in this type of research the result should be the development of theory with a process of clarification.

Having experimented with various types and sizes of audio equipment, each interview was taped using an unobtrusive, flat, 12 inch desktop tape recorder, placed between the research and respondent. Bozett (1980) recognises the ease with which the researcher handles the equipment can be a major influence in its acceptability. This seems to have been a satisfactory arrangement since when asked at the end of the interview, all respondents stated they quickly forgot the tape recorder's presence. Certainly this piece of equipment did not appear to affect the informal atmosphere or the openness with which the respondents answered the questions. Following each interview the researcher wrote down her own thoughts and feelings about the quality of the interview. Some of these notes proved helpful during the analysis phase.

Each interview was then transcribed which proved a time consuming exercise. After much consideration and discussion, it was decided to re-record each original tape using a smaller dictaphone machine. These smaller tapes were then given to an audio typist who transcribed all ten interviews. This was certainly quicker than if the researcher had attempted the transcriptions herself, but it meant listening to the interviews many times in order to become more familiar with the perceptional world of each respondent.

Analysis of data

In order to find out the trained nurses' perceptions of spirituality, a thematic content analysis was carried out on the transcripts. The analysis followed the guidelines set out by Field and Morse (1985) and Burnard (1991), the latter being adapted from Glaser and Strauss' grounded theory approach and from various works on content analysis. The aim was to produce a detailed, systematic recording of themes and issues addressed during the interviews.

The aim of content analysis of text from interview transcripts is to illustrate, through the use of headings and sub-headings, all of the issues that were discussed by respondents during their interviews. Sommer and Sommer (1991) describe content analysis as "a technique for systematically describing the form and content of written or spoken material". Although content analysis can occur at various levels (eg at the level of individual words or at the level of particular phrases), it is probably the case that most nursing researcher's will want to identify key themes or patterns of responses (Berelson 1952, Carney 1982).

Also, it should be borne in mind that research always occurs in a particular context. The researcher never comes to data collection and analysis from a neutral position. The simple analysis of data in the way described here does not account for such context. Alongside the use of the method, the researcher must also consider questions such as: 'what are *my* views on this topic?' and 'why did I ask these particular questions of these particular respondents?' Again, the use of content analysis for its own sake will not suffice. Content analysis merely helps in the ordering of the data that is obtained from a study derived from and devised in a particular social and psychological context. Once content analysis has been carried out, the researcher has to link the findings back to the particular context from which they came.

The method described here offers a rigorous way of grouping together themes in such a way so that *all* of the text contained in a series of interviews is accounted for. Although Sommer and Sommer (1991) suggest that one of the aims of content analysis is *quantification* no attempt is made, with this approach to content analysis, to represent findings in a numerical format - although the method could be adapted for this purpose. In a limited sense, of course, *any* attempt to link sections of text together into categories is a form of quantification.

Following the transcription of the interviews, each was checked with its corresponding tape to ensure accuracy. Corrections were made. Changes in voice and tone, inflections and significance of topics or emotionally charged atmospheres were also noted. Each transcript and tape was therefore reviewed at least 6-8 times to develop an acquaintance with the content and to gain a sense of the thoughts and feelings expressed and hence the respondent's 'whole world'. Rogers (1951) refers to this as the other person's 'frame of reference'. The researcher also referred to her own notes made at the end of each interview.

The first stage of analysis began with open coding. Wilson (1989) defines coding as:

... the process of conceptualizing the underlying patterns of empirical indicators. (Wilson 1989).

Therefore by reading through each line, phrase, paragraph and anecdote in the data and asking what the data was describing, broad general categories appeared. These general categories seemed to emerge from the questions that had been asked during the interview. These were subsequently 'collapsed' into 3 broader 'higher order' headings for convenience: The Concept of Spirituality; Spirituality and Nursing Practice; and The Spirituality of Nurses.

Thus all aspects of the content of the interviews, excluding 'dross', could be described under these 'higher order' headings and the general categories, which included:

- Definitions of spirituality.
- Relevance and importance to the nurse's role.
- Manifestations of patients' spiritual needs.
- Meeting patients' spiritual needs.
- Nurses' beliefs relating to the 'why?' of suffering.
- Nurses' beliefs relating to mortality.
- Nurses' sources of hope and strength.

'Dross' is used by Field and Morse (1985) to describe information that is irrelevant to the issue being discussed which may occur during the interview. However, one of the many difficulties of this type of analysis is having to decide what constitutes such 'dross'.

Each transcript was then read again in order to identify what each person had said under the specific categories. Thus sub headings evolved from the data. At this stage two other people, not involved in the study, were invited to generate their own list of categories and sub headings. Minor adjustments were made.

The sub headings, coded using different highlighter pens, were cut out of the transcripts and all collected together. Multiple photocopies of the transcripts were used in order to ensure that the context of the coded part was maintained. McCracken (1988) notes that everything that is said, is said in a context. Therefore to just cut up words would ignore this fact and thus alter the meaning of what was being said. Furthermore, since all interviews were now cut up into pieces, a complete transcript for each interview was kept for reference. At this stage a validity check was made. A sample of respondents were asked to check the appropriateness of the categories and verify whether what they had said fitted into the categories. Clarification of their statements, phrases etc was also sought.

Once this had been completed the writing up process began. Completed transcripts and original tapes were available and referred to often during this process, in order to check out ambiguities and ensure that the meaning of what was said, was not lost.

Ethical issues

In order to oversee the ethical issues of research in health care, every health authority has an Ethical Committee (Couchman and Dawson 1990). The clinical area which was used in this study was in an authority that only required submission of a research proposal to such a committee if patients were approached. In this study, since no patients were involved, ethical approval was not necessary.

Access to respondents (the trained nurses) was gained formally. Verbal approval was given by the Senior Sister of the clinical area involved and then sought and obtained in writing from the Clinical Nurse Manager and Chief Nurse of the Hospital.

The aim of the research was verbally explained to each of the respondents and their verbal permission to be interviewed sought. In only one case was there a refusal. Once a date and time of interview had been agreed, a letter was given to each confirming the arrangements and explaining once again the purpose of the research.

The aim of requesting access was to ensure everyone knew of the researcher's presence and that the researcher was obtaining data with the respondents' and their manager's informed consent. In addition this appeared to be in keeping with Reason and Rowan (1981) who suggest that researchers in social sciences should be open about their intentions.

Confidentiality is a major concern throughout the documentation of the study. In order to protect the respondents identity, each person was given a random letter a-j. Each respondent is referred to as 'she' throughout the text. Furthermore, the name of the clinical area and hospital has not been identified in order to prevent the respondents being identified locally. It is suffice to know that the clinical area in question is a coronary care unit attached to a medical ward, with staff rotating through both areas.

Objectivity, reliability and validity

Kirk and Miller (1986) note that objectivity is the essential basis of all good research including qualitative designs. They define objectivity as:

> ... the simultaneous realization of as much reliability and validity as possible. Reliability is the degree to which the finding is independent of accidental circumstances of the research, and validity is the degree

to which the finding is interpreted in a correct way (Kirk and Miller 1986).

However, Goodwin and Goodwin (1984) have reported that there is a tendency to ignore reliability and validity or to consider them irrelevant when undertaking research based on a qualitative approach. Nevertheless grounded theory does address such issues (Glaser and Strauss 1967, Stern 1985, Munhall 1989).

Munhall (1989) acknowledges that in qualitative designs, whilst the researcher is a primary instrument, this presence is aimed at coming as close as possible to the reality of the lived experience. The researcher in this study recognised that prior to its commencement she had some degree of knowledge about the concept of spirituality. Indeed this helped formulate the issues and content of the interview schedule. However by laying out her own beliefs, values and perceptions of spirituality, at the beginning of the study and postponing the literature review until the data had been analysed, every effort to acknowledge and lay aside previous preconceptions and biases was made. Ray (1985) refers to this as 'bracketing', the purpose of which is to 'absorb' the experiences as fresh, new and unbiased information. To do this completely proved impossible but the attempt was aimed at ensuring as much reliability and validity as possible.

The researcher was also concerned that her role as tutor to the clinical area may have influenced the respondents' interpretations and descriptions. Every effort was made to create an informal, relaxed, quiet environment, asking open, unbiased questions. In view of the busy, noisy clinical area at the time, each interview was conducted away from the ward, each respondent choosing their own venue. During each interview the researcher attempted to develop a relationship with each respondent and reduce the distance between them.

However, this was balanced with a certain degree of formality. McCracken (1988) argues that the balance between informality and formality is essential if 'rich' reliable data is to be obtained. Not only does a certain amount of formality in speech and demeanour help cast the researcher as someone who asks very personal questions out of, not personal, but professional curiosity but it also helps in reassuring the respondent that the researcher can be trusted to maintain confidentiality. At the same time this degree of formality does not allow intimacy or 'over rapport' to obscure the task in hand.

Two main validity checks were also incorporated into the analysis of the data. Once the interviews had been transcribed and the content categorised, verification of what had been said at interview was sought from three respondents. Ambiguous statements were also clarified. Some minor alterations were made and all stated they were true representations of their perceptions and experiences.

A further validity check was undertaken by asking two colleagues, who were not involved in the study, to independently examine a sample of interview scripts and describe the themes and categories that emerged. On discussion it transpired that similar themes were found, which helped to suggest that the category system had some internal validity.

6 Findings

In this chapter the biographical details of the trained nurses are presented, along with the findings from the analysis of their perceptions of spirituality. These are described under the three broad categories that emerged from the interviews, which were:

- The concept of spirituality
- Spirituality and nursing practice
- The spirituality of nurses

Analysis was also made of an interview with a person who was not a nurse but who worked in a health care situation where spirituality was an important part of the philosophy of care. These findings are presented as a case study. Discussion of these findings will take place along side the presentation. It must be noted that generalisations cannot be made from this study.

Biographical details of the interviewees

There were ten trained nurses interviewed for this study and all worked in a clinical area. Their ages ranged from 21-34 years and their clinical responsibilities depended upon position and grade. Their grades ranged from enroled nurse to senior nurse (a managerial position). The length of time that they had been qualified varied from between 6 months to over 3 years.

The concept of spirituality

Definitions

The first category identified from these interviews was that of definitions of spirituality. Some of these definitions were offered in response to a direct question such as, "How would you define spirituality?" Yet others emerged during the interviews when interviewees were asked to clarify how they were using the term.

The interviewees attempted to define this concept but with varying degrees of ease. Two admitted they found great difficulty in describing and defining the term, whilst another stated:

I've not really thought about it - I'm not a religious person so I'm not that up on what the actual terminology - like spirituality - means. I could never really put a definition on it.

It may have been somewhat unrealistic to ask for a formal definition since we do not often work with 'pure' definitions in every day life. Furthermore, as Rowan (1990) notes, it does appear that one of the difficulties in defining and describing spirituality is its resistance to language.

Religion, faith and culture

Whilst a range of definitions were offered, there was no general agreement as to what constituted spirituality. The most frequently cited definitions related it to religious beliefs, believing in God(s) or Deity and other personal beliefs and faith about life:

It's a belief in God - or God to them.

60

It's a religious belief - a way of life - believing perhaps in one God or more than one God.

It's a religion and a personal thing to believe in.

I think spirituality is just something that somebody believes in - a faith that somebody has.

Probably there's a degree of faith in it even if it's just faith in the people around you.

Two interviewees thought it may also be connected with "culture."

Possibly it's tied up with culture.

I think different religions have different beliefs but we have to be aware of that; and different religions have different ways, different cultures.

Linton, cited by Haralambos (1980), defines the culture of a society, as the way of life of its members, the collection of ideas and habits, learnt and shared and transmitted from generation to generation. Yet for some people, religion is also considered as a way of life. For them it is more than a personal faith/belief (McCavery 1985). For many groups eg. Jews, Hindus, Sikhs and Muslims, cultural restrictions concerning food, recreation and modesty etc are essential components of their religious practices. Since the word spirituality is often equated with the word religion (Kreidler cited by Labun 1988) it is therefore not surprising that the connection between spirituality, religion and culture has been made.

Codes of conduct

Some expanded on these thoughts and considered spirituality as being concerned with the way people lived their lives:

... a code by which people live their lives.

... a driving force, such as the reason and thinking behind how we do things - a code of conduct.

... something that influences the way you think or act or actually live your life - a set of personal values

It rules the way I act with people, the way I run my life .... how I communicate with others.

Words such as "morals" and "ethics" were also used or implied, to provide further elaboration on their initial definitions:

People have certain beliefs, things they believe are right or wrong.

It's to do with things I personally think are wrong and right. These things don't necessarily match up with what other people think are wrong and right or what the Church thinks is wrong or right.

The definition of ethics is fraught with difficulty. The Concise Oxford Dictionary states that it is the 'science of morals' which raises the question 'what is meant by morals?' Tschudin (1986) claims that 'ethics is caring' and that 'to act ethically is to care...to care for ourselves and others'. This approach is certainly attractive to those who claim to be members of caring professions. However in a sense this approach is tautological and gives no real, practical guide to action. Nor can we necessarily assume that 'ethics' and 'caring' are synonyms. Indeed, the advocates of euthanasia often justify their claims to the right to end life, on the basis that they 'care' and wish to relieve suffering, yet many would ask whether such behaviour was ethical. In the place of the last word 'ethical' many people would substitute the word 'right' and it is the consideration of actions, beliefs and attitudes that makes up the study of moral philosophy. In an attempt to decide what is 'right','good', and 'just', Campbell (1975) in trying to separate out the difference between ethics and morals, acknowledged that the Greek and Latin from which the words derive mean roughly the same thing,-'that which is customary or generally accepted, 'but then went on to use the word 'morals' to describe the phenomena which are studied by 'ethics'.

The study of ethics may, therefore, be said to have two aspects, the first is related to how people 'should' behave and is based on the age-old debate engaged in by philosophers as to what is good, right and just, and the second aspect, which can almost be considered to be the opposite side of the same coin, is related to what people actually do and the pressures, personal, cultural, organisational, which influence their action. The first consideration may lead to statements which ignore the consequences, the second sees the result of action as the most important factor.

Thiroux (1980) has established a set of Principles of Ethics which he maintained might be applied to any situation. They are:

- The value of life
- Goodness or rightness
- Justice or fairness
- Truth telling or honesty
- Individual freedom

It is important, according to Thiroux to consider each of these principles when deciding on action. For example, if it is agreed that life is of supreme value, then when is it appropriate to stop striving to maintain it or when is death a realistic option? This is the first principle because without it the others are meaningless. However, Thiroux also states, 'Human beings should revere life and accept death,' which may help in making a decision to turn off a life support system. It may also help remind the nurse that quality of life has to be considered as well as quantity. Yet this fact produces another dilemma, the quality of life enjoyed by a severely handicapped person.may to the healthy young observer, appear to be very low indeed. To the person concerned life may still be precious and worth living. In recent months, there have been court cases which reached the House of Lords about the issue of whether or not quantity of life was as important as quality. Once we move into the domain of judging quality of life, we also move into the difficult area of value judgement.

The question as to the 'goodness' of an action has been debated since Aristotle, with a variety of measures being suggested by which an action may be judged. These range from original intention to the outcome of the activity. Aristotle (see Chase 1925) claimed that virtue lay in the appropriateness of the object or person, for the task, so a 'good knife' is one that is sharp and cuts cleanly, because cutting is the function of a knife. It may also be aesthetically pleasing to look at or in may be ugly, valuable or of little intrinsic worth, but if it does its job, then it is 'good' and produces satisfaction or happiness. At first sight this is an attractive definition and may appear to solve the problem, but closer consideration will reveal some startling difficulties. What, for example, is the purpose of an individual, and can a person be described as' good' because that purpose is met? The shorter

Scottish Catechism states that: 'the chief aim of man is to glorify God and to enjoy Him forever' and Benjamin Disraeli stated that, 'Man...is a being born to believe'. Now whether or not you agree with these statements, or whether you prefer to substitute other functions as the purpose for the existence of human beings, it is easy to see that there may be individuals, perhaps physically or mentally handicapped, or aged and infirm, who may be unable to perform the agreed function. Does this fact make them evil? Obviously not, so that while ability to function appropriately may be a useful way of assessing the value of a knife, it is no help in discussing the value of a man or a woman.

Many people would say that everyone knows what is 'right' and 'good' by the way in which their conscience acts, making them feel that something should, or should not, be carried out. This is not a new idea. Bishop Butler in the 18th century (1926) developed an elaborate theory of conscience in which he claimed that having and obeying a conscience was essential to being classified as human. He explained this by comparing the human personality to a watch, whose separate parts are only of use when placed in relationship to each other. Conscience he claimed, was an essential part of the mechanism of the human personality and without it the individual was incomplete. Further, he claimed that an individual was motivated by three factors. Firstly, by 'particular passions', that is, by basic drives like hunger; some emotional reactions such as fear and anger and 'traits' like shyness or aggression. Secondly, by 'rational calculating principles', which calculate the individual's own long-term happiness, of what Butler called 'cool self love', and the calculation of the happiness of others, which he described as 'the principle of benevolence'; and thirdly, 'conscience' which would hold the superior position and enable the individual to decide between the rightness of action under the other motivating forces. For an individual to disobey his or her conscience, according to Butler, was to destroy the natural balance of their personality.

All this sounds fine, but of course people do not always obey their conscience. Another difficulty is that my conscience may say one thing and in an identical situation yours may dictate another. Indeed, it is this very conflict which causes so many problems in nursing/medical practice. One person fully believes that it is wrong to destroy life in any situation and therefore their conscience forbids them to assist with abortion; another believes, equally vehemently, that there are occasions when abortion is appropriate. Both must follow their own conscience and thus no consensus can be reached. Instead, to use Sartre's (1948) words:

the individual is entirely alone and abandoned in his decision; he, and he alone, must take the responsibility.

Another approach taken by a number of people when deciding on a course of action is to consider whether or not they would like it done to them. Charles Kingsley (1869) used this principle in his book *The Water Babies* when he developed the character Mrs Do-as -you-would-be-done-by. Kant (1785) developed this point of view but also said that morality was doing one's duty for duties sake. He described a series of actions as 'Categorical imperatives' that is, they must be followed. These are:

- So act that the maxim of your action can become a universal law for all rational beings.
- Act as if the maxim of your action were to become by your will a universal law of nature.
- So act as to treat humanity, whether in your own person or in that of any other, in every case as an end, never as a mere means.

However, there are problems in applying this law of 'universality' when dealing with people who are themselves different and thus require different consideration. Does a commitment to preserve life mean that every patient who dies must be resuscitated because that is the universal law? Some would argue 'yes', while many would want to say 'it all depends'. Indeed, some would wish the patient to be given the opportunity to request that resuscitation should, or should not be carried out, for, if this choice is denied, the patient may be used as a 'means' to enable the nursing or medical staff to comfort themselves with the thought that everything had been done for the patient. Yet Kant said that the person must be an 'end in himself'. Consider the arguments used to support the decision to spend money in one area of health care rather than another. Remarks such as 'he is so young' or 'she is old and had her life'. Heart transplants before treatment for arthritis, acute care before chronic, and so on. In all these statements 'ends' are implied regarding the worth of the individual in relation to their likely contribution to society: means, not ends in themselves.

More acceptable may be the consideration of whether or not an action produces happiness. Philosophers known as utilitarians who may be represented by Jeremy Bentham and John Stuart Mill, assert that what is good is pleasure and happiness and what is bad is pain. A good action, therefore, is one that produces more pleasure than pain. However as any parent will know often a child's wishes have to be denied, thus producing unhappiness, because granting the request may be dangerous for the child. Can such a denial be considered bad? A further problem is that happiness for one group may produce unhappiness for another. Who is to be satisfied? The one with most power? So develops the tyranny of the majority.

From this discussion, it is obvious that it is difficult (perhaps impossible) to formulate one rule by which every situation may be judged, so that it can be said with certainty, 'this action is good, right and just.' One common thread running throughout the debate is the conviction that people cannot be treated as a collection of things such as knives and that each person has to be regarded individually. Indeed this is one of the first lessons learnt by the new entrant to nursing. All patients must be treated alike.

Even this statement may be contentious: discussion as to whether an action is just or fair cannot stop at saying that all must be treated alike when it is quite clear that all are not the same to start with. Is discrimination, positive or negative, ever justified? We have already considered the problem in relation to expenditure on health care for specific groups. There is an apparent paradox in the statements 'all people must be treated alike' and yet 'each person has to be treated as an individual'. This paradox can be easily resolved, the nurse must not differentiate between patients on the grounds of colour, social class, education, attractiveness of personality and so, only on the basis of the activity required to meet the patient's individual needs. However, this does not help the decision as to how to allocate scarce resources.

Schrock (1980) claims that nurses are often less than honest in their dealings with patients, yet honesty and truthfulness make up Thiroux's fourth principle. Most people in everyday life support varying degrees of honesty and truth telling. So much is this accepted that the telling of a 'white lie' carries little stigma on the basis that to do so may be kind. Can this ever really be justified? To what extent is the 'whole truth' necessary? Difficult questions, especially when caring for some patients, nevertheless a principle of morality.

Finally, the principle of individual freedom. This, if present, will influence the way the first four principles are held and acted upon. What is more, it implies autonomy of action so that no one else can be held responsible for the actions of another. Nurses frequently question to what extent they have autonomy and, therefore, whether they can be held responsible for the care they give. Codes of Conduct assume that the individual is accountable, but to what extent are they correct?

What all this apparently leads to is a belief that a moral basis for action has to be rooted in the perception of the intrinsic worth of the individual and that persons right to self determination. (Christians would back up this respect by explaining that man is created in the image of God.) The debate as to what constitutes a person has already been touched upon. Most agree that the definition includes the possession of an individual with humanoid characteristics; with a capacity, however small, to communicate and be communicated with (not necessarily by speech). 'Respect of person' in this context, requires activity which is a combination of both rational and emotional elements used in a relationship of involvement with other individuals, so that their wishes, thoughts and aspirations are taken into account.

This approach, the respect of persons, has some important implications. First, there is no final set of moral rules to guide action, as modification may have to take place in the light of the individual; secondly, the individual is given greater value than society; thirdly, it demands an attempt to maintain an ongoing relationship with the individual, so that the person does not become an object to whom things are done.

Seedhouse (1988) states that ethics and morals are words whose significance and meaning enter into all areas of human thought and action. Tschudin's (1986) distinction between the two words is that morals usually refers to sexuality and religious dogma and ethics refers to broader issues and ideals. However both appear to refer to the individual character of a person and also to ways of human behaviour.

The words are also concerned not only with how people 'should' live their lives ie. what is good, right or just but also with what people 'actually do.' The former deals with the 'consequences' of action and the latter, the 'result' of the action. Thus in drawing up any personal code of conduct both aspects need to be considered. It would appear that ethics and morals play an important part in guiding peoples behaviour. Thus definitions encompassing such terms as ethics, morals and codes of conduct, can be favourably compared to Ellerhorst-Ryan's (1985) definition of spirituality - the central philosophy of life which guides peoples' conduct.

Dimension of an individual

Spirituality was also identified as being part of the individual:

A sub-conscious state.

67

Something that's important - very close to you.

Spirituality is very much part of my make-up, it's part of my personality. It forms my life with people, how I communicate, what vibes I give off .... it's what I think about life after death, how I feel about God and my mortality .... it's there all the time and it's reassuring to know I have a sense of spirituality. ... it is there in every one, nobody's made up of only hearts and kidneys, it's there but unfortunately some people haven't had to look into themselves.

Indeed two interviewees recognised a connection between the spiritual and the psychological aspect of the person.

It is certainly not something physical - there's a lot of emotion involved in it.

It is how people mentally deal with problems and things that happen in their lives - how they perceive things that happen in the world.

There is acknowledgement of the difficulty in differentiating the psychosocial dimension of the person with the spiritual dimension (Highfield and Cason 1983, Piles 1990). But whilst they are inextricably intertwined, the spiritual dimension appears to encompass something more. If, as already noted, Fish and Shelly, cited by Peterson (1985), suggest that the spiritual component of the person helps answer some of the questions that occur as a result of life experiences and traumas, then it would seem that "how people mentally deal with problems" would be an appropriate description of the spiritual dimension of the person.

The case study also considered spirituality as part of the self:

The inner need that we all have... finding an inner peace.

She described her own personal experiences of finding this inner peace:

Up to the age of 36 years, I hadn't recognised what that inner need was... But there was always an unfulfilled need and a need that made me feel guilty at times because I couldn't quite put my finger on why I wasn't as happy as I should have been, having a happy marriage and nice home, two lovely children. So I should have had everything but there was just something missing and I never knew what it was until I found my own spirituality within me and that fulfilled the need.

In contrast to the other definitions, for this person spirituality appeared to be not only an important dimension of the person but a state of mind. Once found, she felt an "inner peace". This seems to suggest a sense of inner harmony and the presence of spiritual well being, an aspect of spirituality not specifically highlighted by the nurses. It could be argued that if the trained nurses had achieved 'wholeness' and 'spiritual health' then they too would have been able to describe spirituality in such terms. But to do this would make too many assumptions about their spiritual integrity.

A more likely explanation would be that the nurses had not developed a certain level of consciousness about themselves. Heron (1988) speaks of this as the 'higher intuitive self,' the 'transpersonal self,' the 'cosmic self.' Unless individuals have undergone such experiences or something like, finding an 'inner peace,' or meeting a 'deeper self,' such descriptions seem hard to follow and somewhat nonsensical.

What does it mean to talk about 'the self'? There are spatial difficulties here: where is the self? Is it part of our physical make up? Is it something spiritual? Is it something separate to the body and if so, what is its *relationship* to the body? Questions like these have interested philosophers and theologians for centuries but these issues have also been of interest to social scientists.

The existential school of philosophy discussed the issue under the heading of 'ontology': the study of *being* (Macquarrie 1972). To talk of the self, for the existentialists, is to talk of something more than just bodily existence. It is to describe the fact of being a conscious, knowing human being. It must be noted, however, that any notion of 'self' must also clearly be rooted in a *physical* existence. At the same time, Sartre (1948) is involved in Cartesian dualism and consciously splitting of the mind from the body, by his own admission. Sartre's discussion of self is necessarily a *psychological* one. Of the more recent commentators on the question of mind, Searle seems to clear this particular hurdle well when he suggests that minds are a product of brains: a mental event is necessarily also a physical one (Searle 1983). Thus, if the self and spirituality are in some ways the same thing, we are left to wonder if spirituality might be a 'physical' thing.

The case study's awareness arose when she was given a book following the death of her grandmother:

So I read the book and I realised there was a whole load of questions that this book didn't ask and it set me on a search. At this point I didn't even know I was looking for spirituality but I did start looking for answers to our reason to be and what life was all about. It only came about some months later ... when I really got into looking and seeking the truth and opening up the spiritual aspect...it's like a flower opening...

She concluded however, by recognising that such experiences and such an awareness could never be "forced" on others:

It happens to them because it is right for them not because I'm telling them about me...

Whilst some nurses admitted they had not thought about spirituality before, the researcher gained the impression from all the nurses that they had not given much consideration to the concept before agreeing to be interviewed. Many hesitated for several minutes before answering these questions or prefixed their responses with "I'm not sure but...", "That's a difficult one..." Developing an awareness of their own spirituality may not have been addressed before. This issue of self awareness will be discussed again at a later stage.

Summary

Generalisations cannot be drawn from these interviews but the varying definitions of spirituality, given by these trained nurses and the case study, do appear to support the literature's recognition of the complexity of spirituality and its unique interpretation by individuals.

This is of significance to nurse education. If spirituality involves such broad issues as religion, culture, beliefs about life, ethics and morals, and self awareness, it seems unrealistic to expect to increase nurses' understanding about spirituality in a single session.

However, if a nursing curriculum encompasses such core themes as ethics and morals, self awareness and adopts a multicultural approach to belief systems, then educating nurses about such a concept appears a more feasible option. It is hoped that with the adoption and implementation of the proposals of Project 2000 (UKCC 1987) that such curricula are now in existence, so enabling spirituality to be integrated into nurse education rather than being an isolated and often misunderstood concept.

Spirituality and nursing practice

Relevance and importance to the nurses' role

All interviewees believed the notion of spirituality to be important and relevant to the role of the nurse, with a small number prefixing important with "very" or "extremely".

Reasons

The reasons for this relevance varied. For one nurse it was because of the importance of the spiritual dimension of the person:

> *I think it's extremely important because it's a vital part of people whether it's a religious need or just the basic needs and beliefs that people have that affect the way they think or the way their illness affects them. It's something that has to be addressed. I think it's an integral part of you.*

Another felt meeting patients' spiritual needs was part of the nurses' role:

> *I don't think we fully understand or take into account patients needs. But it's part of the nurses' role to meet spiritual needs, it's part of actual recovery really.*

Interestingly, the case study also made reference to recovery when discussing the importance of spirituality in her health care situation:

> *Without it I think it's rare that somebody would really make a good recovery because we are leaving out the essential part of ourselves. Most healing goes on as far as I understand at that deepest level. It filters through all the different levels of our being until it gets to the physical. There is no reason for the physical to be out of balance if you have every part of you in balance.*

Yet for another nurse its importance and relevance was felt on a personal level. She believed spirituality to be:

... an integral part of my job. I can't believe I could do it properly or adequately at all if I didn't have spiritual beliefs... I think if I didn't have any spiritual beliefs it would be very difficult to take a person as a whole and feel empathy with them.

The importance of treating people as individuals was an explanation given by two other nurses:

I think everyone has got to respect one another's beliefs whether you agree with them or not... We've got to observe as much as we can, what people individually want.

I just think it's important to take everybody as an individual and abide by what their needs are.

Extent of nurses' consideration of spirituality

There were also a small number of nurses who voluntarily commented on the extent of nurses' consideration of spirituality in the clinical area:

It's generally done quite poorly.

I don't know really that we do cater properly for it.

On the same theme, another noted more generally:

I don't think it's of prime importance in nursing today.

Whilst for another it was not seen as a priority:

It's not one of the main things that we think about when we care for patients.

This is in keeping with our previous suggestion that it seems likely that a number of people to not consider the spiritual domain at all - as nurses or as patients. Two nurses tried to find some kind of explanation for their comments. For one it was "poor understanding" and the other:

... because a lot of us don't necessarily think about it ourselves.

The literature available on nursing and spirituality would perhaps lead to the expectation that the nurses would be aware of the importance/relevance of spirituality to the nurse's role. However, the extent of the nurses' appreciation of the dichotomy between this awareness and its incorporation into nursing practice was not anticipated.

The reasons offered by the two nurses for this lack of incorporation suggest further education about spirituality may go some way in dealing with this dichotomy. Indeed, this need for better training and further education has already been identified in several studies (Highfield and Cason 1983, Simsen 1986, Edwardson 1988 and Piles 1990).

Nevertheless, even if the education and training about spirituality were to be improved, it would not guarantee the integration of theory and practice. Whilst the future of nursing and the welfare of patients demands a narrowing of the gap between the educational ideals and the clinical reality (Copcutt 1984), there appears to be a danger of building up a body of knowledge in nursing unrelated to the actual practice of nursing. Furthermore, this gap between the educational ideal and the clinical reality is one of the major causes of dissatisfaction in nursing (Smith 1981). Yet if nurses themselves are able to truly understand the relevance and importance of such a concept, this incorporation into nursing practice may go some way to being achieved. In any educational programme it is suggested that adequate time should be given to discussing such matters of relevance and importance.

Manifestations of patients' spiritual needs

When the nurses were asked to describe patients' spiritual needs, all acknowledged that they had encountered such patients. However, the descriptions of these needs varied.

Groups of patients

Examples of the patients who had been in their care were given as "terminally ill" or the "dying person" or "a hindu, muslim or somebody that would be a little bit different."

With the elderly, you get a lot of people thinking about their bereaved wife and wanting to be with their bereaved wife thinking they are going to another world to be with them.

Religious/cultural manifestations

Some of the nurses identified spiritual needs as "religious needs" or gave religion based answers:

Anybody wanting to take communion or the vicar coming in from home.

Some patients maybe want to go to Church on Sunday. If they can't make it to Church on the Sunday they would like to have communion on the ward.

Catholics wanting to see the Priest.

Others identified more cultural aspects. "Special diets","meditation time", needs relating to "washing and praying", and particularly needs/practices to be observed "following death." One nurse highlighted a spiritual need of hindus:

They need a lot of family input into their care.

However she then reflected on this and wondered whether this was more an emotional need.

Some nurses also highlighted individual experiences with particular patients to help clarify their answers:

One lady who couldn't have a bath - a Muslim - wanted a wash under running water so we sat her in an inch of water and we poured water from a jug...... Another patient, again I don't know what religion he was but he had an eating hand and a washing hand they tried to fix his eating hand with a drip a board and bandage, the therefore didn't eat. He didn't speak English.

A canon and his wife who was terminally ill, so they spent a lot of time together. He obviously had a deep belief in God.

... a few people I can remember have actually talked about dying and have expressed fears or just very rational views and want to get things organised for their deaths, for the family; so spirituality definitely comes into play here. The people who wanted to talk about death may express emotions of any sort... Occasionally I have had God come into the conversation if someone is very ill or when talking to a relative of a sick person.

It was perhaps not surprising that the examples given were mostly related to religion or culture. However, as the literature has highlighted, these are only some of the ways people develop and express their spiritual needs. Unless nurses recognise the many different expressions, there is a danger that this dimension of the person will be neglected.

Other manifestations

Nevertheless, not all the nurses gave religious or cultural examples. For one nurse, patients' spiritual needs were recognised by:

Possibly being anxious, sharp, cross, or not wanting to co-operate.

It could be said that the examples this nurse gave were not needs but problems. However the nurse continued:

I would see these as spiritual needs because it is something that really is affecting them, their life style. It's not physical so you would approach it in a totally different way but it's not religious-based needs at all; but it's perhaps something I could help with.

Another nurse commented:

Some believe spiritual needs are religious beliefs but they are not always or quite often they are not. Some patients want to discuss dying and that sort of thing. They just want to talk. This happens a lot at night.

Whilst these descriptions give a selection of manifestations of spiritual needs, they do not appear to identify the specific spiritual needs, common to all individuals. As already noted in the literature review these include, the need to give and receive love (O'Brien 1982, Highfield and Cason 1983, Peterson 1985). Yet they were acknowledged, to some extent, by the case study:

> *I suppose our needs are all the same and there isn't anybody that has a different need than another in the spiritual sense and wanting to become whole, wanting to make that connection with ourselves, a deeper inner connection. But we try to fulfil that need perhaps in different and more earthy ways. We may become obsessed about something and put our heart and passion into something.*

However it would seem that the realisation that spiritual needs are common to everyone, is fundamental in acknowledging the spiritual dimension of all individuals. It is how individuals meet their spiritual needs and the extent of their recognition by nurses that are diverse. Because spiritual needs involve so many different and complex aspects, problems and difficulties may be encountered during the assessment process.

Meeting patients' spiritual needs

Assessment methods

When asked about how they met patients' spiritual needs, most nurses felt that this began with the initial admission and assessment process.

This included assessment of particular needs, "eating", "socialising", "hygiene". The use of Roper's Activities of Living Model of Care was highlighted by one nurse. However for many nurses, spiritual assessment involved specifically asking about their patients' religion. Only a small proportion of these followed this up, by finding out whether they were practising or not. For example:

> *It tends to start with the admission process and when admitting people I would try not just asking "What religion are you?" but perhaps go a little bit deeper. Were they practising? Would they find it beneficial to see the relevant Minister? This sort of thing. You can tell if it doesn't seem too important to them and I would leave it there. But if they show an interest in that sort of question then I would take it as far as I could and offer perhaps visits from the Chaplains.*

For two nurses, questioning went beyond religion:

Finding out about their religion and their beliefs on life/death.

... finding out about them generally, what they do, what they do with their time, reading, walking, it can give you a rough idea of what they are like as a person and if they are quite emotional, and also how they speak about their illness for example 'it could be worse nurse'; what sort of attitude they have towards their illness. All this can give a clue as to their spirituality.

The approach towards spiritual assessment was recognised by some of the nurses as being important:

I would make sure I'd sus them out first before I go barging in with religion... obviously I don't push them.

I wouldn't come straight out with anything blunt. I'd ask what they did at home, if they had any hobbies and see what they say. If they said they were involved in the Church I might ask what do they do, who they are friendly with and then perhaps lead onto 'Is there anything that we can do whilst you are not at home, anybody we can contact?'

Whilst this study demonstrated that these nurses used no structured format for spiritual assessment, other than asking about their patients' religion, it does highlight that this aspect of care was not totally neglected.

Difficulties related to assessment

However as Peterson and Nelson (1987) note, for spiritual assessment to be restricted to questions, particularly just a few about religion, is unsatisfactory. The literature review has already highlighted the need to consider observational and listening skills as well as other types of questions to elicit information about the spiritual dimension of patients (Shelley 1982, Carson 1989c).

Yet it may be that the use of the spiritual history guides suggested by Stoll (1979) and O'Brien (1982) are unrealistic in the clinical areas. Such a point was raised by some trained nurses during a recent session about spirituality led by the researcher. They felt such questions were an intrusion into a person's privacy. This supports one of Granstrom's (1985) reasons for nurses' reluctance to become involved in spiritual aspects of care.

This unsatisfactory approach to spiritual assessment may therefore have something to do with the nurses' feelings about discussing spiritual concerns. Indeed in this study, some nurses admitted finding it difficult initiating conversation about spiritual matters. This was for several reasons:

Because I don't have any religious beliefs myself.

You never know what the reaction is going to be.

I think it's hard really... I think the majority of people don't really think about their spirituality and I don't think they understand what their own spiritual needs are. I mean, if you asked me what mine were I don't think I'd know.

Interestingly more nurses felt less "uncomfortable" about responding to patients when they talked about their spiritual needs than if they had to initiate conversation on the same topic. However one nurse commented:

But some people may feel threatened when people start expressing spirituality on other people, especially those with strong religious beliefs.

Although another nurse, who had strong religious beliefs stated:

When someone is very ill, or when someone has died, it is very difficult to console them and sometimes I do try to bring God into that conversation, but I understand that this is very difficult and sensitive if someone has just lost somebody and a righteous nurse comes along... but occasionally it has worked and consoled them and I feel that if I can share my belief in God while we're here then perhaps I can help somebody in their hour of need as it were, then I have done some good in representing my faith.

These feelings also support Granstrom's (1985) ideas about the reasons behind nurses' reluctance to become involved in spiritual aspects - fear and concern about patients' reactions; fear and concern about being threatened by the strong religious beliefs of others; lack of clarity of nurses' own belief systems and lack of spiritual awareness. Yet if nurses are to be committed to helping patients, in all aspects, including the spiritual dimension, they need to address these issues and increase their knowledge and understanding of such matters. This has implications for nurse education. In addition it may suggest that nurses' own belief systems could have some influence on their interaction with patients. This point will be discussed again at a later stage.

Spiritual care

It seemed that for most nurses, offering visits by the Chaplain/Priest or appropriate religious minister, was the main way of meeting patients' spiritual needs. However for others, contact with religious leaders was only offered if the nurses felt they could not deal with the needs or issues being discussed. Family involvement was also cited by some as an important part of spiritual care.

Examples of such care were given:

It was dinner time and the Chaplain came round and we delayed dinner until she (the patient) had finished communion.

We ordered a vegetarian dinner from the kitchen, also we let the family bring in food.

As Wilson-Barnett (1985) notes, admission to hospital is stressful and when this hospitalisation is sudden, as in critical illness, it has been described as a 'crisis' (Molter 1979). Yet as Miller (1991) notes, patients rarely experience 'crisis' on their own. More often than not it is also experienced by those with whom they are close, often their family.

When surrounded by a strange environment, families also experience feelings of loneliness associated with the physical and psychological separation from the patient (King and Gregor 1984), the need for hope (Molter 1979) and feelings of anger, helplessness and uncertainties about the future, all of which suggest a degree of spiritual distress. Spiritual care may therefore be of help, not only to the patients, but to their families as well.

Necessary skills

Interpersonal skills were also recognised by many as being significant in meeting patients' spiritual needs. "Talking with patients", "questioning", "listening", "picking up clues", as was the type of atmosphere for discussing such issues:

Trying to provide an atmosphere in which they (the patients) feel comfortable in what they want to express.

Furthermore there was recognition of spending enough time with the patients:

It's something you do have to listen to (ie.spiritual needs). You've got to give time and space and if you can't give your time, then you must say you will come back and do go back.

One nurse identified the need to separate nurses' and patients' spiritual beliefs:

I certainly wouldn't offer any of my beliefs because I don't think that's relevant at all and I think it might inhibit what they were going to say.

Another acknowledged the importance of respecting patients' views:

I would respect anything that is important to somebody else because if they are important to somebody else then you have to treat it as though it exists.

Counselling

Patterson and Pepinsky, cited by Dobson (1987), have explained counselling as a non judgemental relationship, allowing patients to seek solutions to their own problems in a listening, caring environment and these descriptions by the nurses, seem to recognise some of the qualities that would be essential for such a relationship eg. time, listening, valuing patients' views.

Empathy is another necessary quality. Burnard (1989) describes empathy as the ability, more or less, to enter fully into the world of the patient, so requiring the nurse to attempt to view the world from the patient's point of view. Whilst Rogers (1987) notes that the degree to which such empathy can develop is open to debate, it does seem essential to attempt to develop a degree of mutual understanding.

Empathy was not specifically mentioned by the nurses but the researcher felt that this type of understanding was implicit rather than explicit in some of the descriptions of the discussions with patients.

We (the patient and I) just talked about life and after life and tried to work out what it (life) all means.

One nurse had observed and discussed with one of her patients how he had met his own spiritual needs in the clinical area:

He thought that his needs were met by people being kind to him and people being kind to other patients. He saw it in the way by which nurses on the ward were being kind, perhaps offering a drink to someone when they didn't ask for it.

This experience made this particular nurse realise that spiritual care was not purely based on religion:

... because people's views and ideas are totally different and everybody needs to be treated as an individual.

.... part of it is communication and getting to know what the patients actually feel and obviously that's from talking to them.... Talking to them even when you are doing something else, perhaps if you are helping them to have a wash or whatever; you don't have to actually sit down and chat. I think in effect it's probably better to do it like that because people are more open than if you sit down and actually say "Right, come on let's talk about it".

The researchers are aware of the difficulty in defining spiritual care per se. It is often too easy to emphasise the 'doing aspect' eg. calling on the Chaplain, making arrangements for communion, rather than the 'being with' or 'being there' aspect. Yet some of these descriptions do emphasise the importance of 'presence'. As Ersser (1991) notes, mere companionship from a caring person may be reassuring in itself. More often than not, just being available is of more significance to the spiritually distressed person than anything that can be said or done. Kubler Ross (1969) talks about facing death and considers that 'healthy acceptance' usually only occurs when patients have been encouraged to express their feelings and emotions eg. anger, rage, crying, to someone who can quietly sit and listen.

Counselling skills recommended by nurses, for nurses, are usually of the client-centred variety. The term 'client-centred', first used by Carl Rogers (1951) refers to the notion that it is the client, himself, who is best able to decide how to find the solutions to their problems in living. 'Client-centred', in this sense may be contrasted with the idea of 'counsellor-centred' or 'professional-centred', both of which may suggest that someone other than the client is the 'expert'. Whilst this may be true when applied to certain concrete 'factual' problems: housing, surgery, legal problems and so forth, it is difficult to see how it can apply to personal life issues. In such cases, it is the client who identifies the problem and the client who, given time and space, can find their way through the problem to the solution. Murgatroyd (1985) summarises the client-centred position as follows:

- a person in need has come to your for help
- in order to be helped they need to know that you have understood how they think and feel
- they also need to know that, whatever your own feelings about who or what they are or about what they have or have not done, you accept them as they are
- you accept their right to decide their own lives for themselves
- in the light of this knowledge about your acceptance and understanding of them they will begin to open themselves to the possibility of change and development
- but if they feel that their association with you is conditional upon them changing, they may feel pressurised and reject your help.

These guidelines may be particularly appropriate in the field of spiritual counselling in nursing in that they are not dogmatic and allow for the patient to think and talk through his or her own beliefs and values. Within the client-centred approach to counselling there is no place for proselytising or evangelising for a particular point of view or for a particular set of religious beliefs and, given the current emphasis on patient-centred care, this would seem to be in line with modern approaches to thinking about nursing interventions.

Confidentiality

Passing on relevant information about meeting patients' needs raised issues about confidentiality. Handover time at shift change over provided an opportunity for some to discuss this information, to ensure everything was done to fulfil these needs. However, some were conscious of the type of information patients had divulged to the nurses:

This is quite private information.

Things that they tell you might be quite personal.

But this nurse continued by stating:

... but by just allowing him to talk might help him at that moment... the interaction between two people is enough rather than the whole world knowing.

For patients to confide in nurses there has to be a degree of trust. Baly (1983) states that nurses do not inspire this by their cleverness but by their integrity and honour as people. Tschudin (1986) argues, in pursuing greater professionalism for nursing, nurses cannot foster more confidence and trust by never revealing any confidential matter, as this may hinder care. However breaking a confidence may be doing the same. How nurses decide to act with such information will depend on the relationship the patients and nurses have. But to judge correctly when to act on such information will depend on the nurses' ability to really hear what their patients have said.

Healing

Although working in a health care situation, the case study was not involved in any assessment of spiritual needs or delivery of care. However she considered that the key to meeting people's spiritual needs was through "healing."

It was not the purpose of this study to explore in detail this particular intervention. Yet there appears a growing appreciation of this complementary approach to medicine (Green 1986, Beeny 1990, Benor 1991). However many doctors disagree about whether the spiritual dimension has any relevance to their work with patients, as it cannot be defined in scientific terms.

'Healing' includes such therapies as therapeutic touch, laying on of hands (Benor 1991) and Green (1986) considers that:

A well ordered healing ritual with the laying on of hands, peaceful accepting atmosphere and great emphasis on love, 'oneness' and completeness can be a first class antidote to stress, fear and loneliness, thus freeing and mobilising the body's natural healing and calming, healing the mind and spirit (Green 1986).

It is interesting to note that the kind of atmosphere it is hoped to create during 'healing' also has strong similarities to the kind of atmosphere necessary for the caring approach it is suggested nurses adopt in order to give spiritual care.

The concept of healing appears in both the medical and the spiritual literature. It is interesting to note, in passing, that some doctors may claim to 'heal' whilst the concept is also firmly rooted in certain aspects of the church and, in this context, it is to be supposed that God 'does' the healing.

Summary

Whilst there seemed an awareness of the relevance and importance of the concept of spirituality to the role of the nurse, there was also an appreciation that the spiritual dimensions of people were not always addressed in clinical practice.

On the whole spiritual needs were confined to particular groups of patients and related to religious or cultural needs. Furthermore there seemed little recognition that spiritual needs were common to all, let alone any acknowledgement of the spiritual needs of patients admitted to hospital with acute illnesses such as myocardial infarctions.

Conclusions could be drawn that spirituality was somewhat of a neglected aspect of care. Indeed reasons were offered as to why the concept of spirituality was not considered. Furthermore it seemed that no structured assessment was used by the nurses, although it must be noted that some nurses did identify 'interventions' that could be described as essential components of spiritual care.

No generalisations can be drawn from this study but it suggests that the nurses require more knowledge and greater understanding about spirituality and nursing practice. This has implications for nurse education. Any educational programme about spirituality should carefully consider its content and include such topics as relevance and importance to nursing practice, methods of spiritual assessment and the development of essential skills required for spiritual care.

The spirituality of nurses

An initial assumption was made that the majority of the nurses being interviewed would not have considered their own spiritual dimension in any depth before and as such would not have really examined their own beliefs or discovered the principles, religious or non religious, by which their lives were guided. To ask directly about their spirituality or their belief system seemed inappropriate. Therefore in order to gain some insight into their spiritual dimension, questions were asked relating to a variety of issues, as suggested by Stoll (1979) and Jacik (1989). These were thoughts and feelings about suffering; the meaning and purpose of life and mortality; the meaning of God; the significance of religion; and sources of love, hope and strength.

Beliefs and convictions relating to the 'why?' of suffering

The responses to this question appeared to fall into two main categories. Those answering in fairly practical terms and those who offered more philosophical explanations.

Pragmatic explanations

One nurse put herself in the patient's place and tried to relate to how she would feel with:

I try and think how I would feel in every aspect of it. The loss of control, the feeling that you are not in control, people talking over you, making decisions for you. I think of the things that would irritate me about it and I try and make sure that it doesn't happen...because if there is something pain or whatever they shouldn't be like that, there is no reason and we're supposed to take a problem solving approach

*into things like that, so we should actually be looking for the solution
not just the 'why's'.*

In addition she looked to nursing for explanations as to why someone was
suffering eg. "lack of information", "ineffective communication", "poor pain
control."

Two other nurses also took somewhat of a practical approach. This was
clearly explained by one of them:

> *I think, well let's get on with the situation and try and do your best to
> make the patients as comfortable as possible, rather than pondering on
> the 'why?'*

Although both nurses admitted they had not "sat down and thought about
suffering like this before", one of them felt that her feelings may have been
influenced by her upbringing:

> *.... the way I was taught to think of things. It was always what can we
> do about it rather than 'why?'*

Philosophical explanations

For other nurses, seeing suffering made them question God's existence and
purpose.

> *I wonder if there really is a God, why would he let people suffer so
> much. But I can't really find an answer to the question.*

> *I find it quite hard to come to terms with sometimes. If there is a God,
> why is he letting people go through this?*

Some nurses felt that whilst they had considered this question before, they
could not come up with any definite answers. Nevertheless they implied that
there was a certain degree of injustice involved. One commented:

> *That's a difficult question isn't it? I don't know really. I do think about
> it because my father was quite young when he died and you think, well,
> why did it happen to him, why not to someone else? I don't think there
> are any answers for it.*

One nurse appeared to have thought about this issue in some detail and gave examples of working with different types of patients. The issue about 'why certain people suffer' had arisen for her when caring for children:

> *I still find I can't answer that question 'why does a child have to suffer or die? but then I go one step further and believe that there is a place for them and a job for them to do somewhere else.... but with adults I don't tend to ask 'why?' because they are older; they have experienced many happy years of living with their families and they seem more accepting... then the older they get, the more difficult it becomes, when you see an elderly relative left behind after 70 years of happy marriage or whatever when they're left alone. It is very upsetting but they've had a good life ...*

Nevertheless she felt that more consideration should be given to this issue:

> *If everyone was honest about their feelings relating to illness and suffering and could talk about it, it may be the question 'why?' wouldn't come up. I tend to think 'why not?'*

The case study appeared to have given this some consideration before. There was an element of acceptance in her tone and explanation. Suffering seemed somewhat inevitable but would get easier with each life:

> *Only when you've really looked into this and come to a really good understanding to what life is all about can you answer this question... My own belief is that we have many, many lives, different bodies but with the essence within us. We therefore come again and again until we become so perfected we don't need to come again.*

Nurses are brought into close contact with suffering and they are more often than not the group of professionals to whom patients look for support in relation to their anxieties about illness, their physical discomfort or spiritual distress.

However as McGilloway (1985b) notes, given that nurses, despite their 'acquired culture' and training belong to a wider society, it would be strange if they were altogether exempt from the kinds of emotional reactions of ordinary people to illness and suffering situations. James (1989) a nurse sociologist, spent five months as a participant observer in a hospice and described how patients' emotions such as grief, anger, loss, despair and frustration were not only distressing to watch but were awkward to respond to. Indeed the nurses sometimes chose to concentrate on the physical aspects of patient care in order to avoid the difficult relationships and become too emotionally involved.

Such defence mechanisms allow care givers to confine their reciprocal interactions to certain limits, while at the same time offering protection against feelings of grief for their patients' suffering. It may be that by not considering the 'why?' of suffering, nurses are providing themselves with another distancing device. Yet by addressing such an issue themselves, nurses may become more attuned to their patients' spiritual dimension and feel less threatened when patients consider their own suffering and question their existing beliefs.

Meaning and purpose of life

Some of the nurses stated they could come to no definite conclusions about the meaning and purpose of life, whilst others admitted they had not given the question a great deal of consideration before. One wondered if this was because of her lack of life experiences:

> *I don't really have any strong convictions or beliefs. I'd rather be open minded to whatever there is around... I am open to all possibilities, there has got to be something... I think my coping mechanism is to deal with it rather than just sit and pull my hair out and 'bawl' about it and analyse it.*

The case study noted that her beliefs about the meaning and purpose of life had developed over time:

> *I would say it evolved over some years now - about nine years. You don't just read one or two books and think 'yes this is my truth!'... Conviction comes from within yourself and that takes a few years, through all sorts of experiences.*

Other nurses however attempted to explain their beliefs, although it was apparent that most had not considered this question before. Many paused for some time before answering or began with such statements as:

That's a tough one. The meaning of life? I don't really know but...

They then proceeded to give some kind of explanation, working through their ideas as they talked them through. For example:

I don't know really .... I think if you have any trauma or actual upset in your life, it makes you a stronger person when you come out of it the other side. I think things are sent to try us and that people have things to cope with and it makes them a better person at the end of the day.

One nurse felt she had some kind of meaning and purpose in her life:

I'd like to think that I'm here for a purpose, not just to have a good time and get the most out of life and people. I believe there is a heaven. I don't know in what way it is going to present itself but I strongly believe that the spirit goes on. When I say this to some people they laugh but I believe the body remains and decays but the spirit is much stronger and the spirit helps those who are left on earth, the way they come to terms with things, how they react in their life. I'd like to think it was the spirit that was doing that. So I don't believe we all end when our physical bodies give up on us... I think I've served a certain degree of purpose in my nursing and I feel that I am doing some good in my job. I have a desire, in my nursing career, to prove something, achieve something and make a little mark somewhere along the line in the nursing profession.

It appears that to find meaning in nursing is of significance. Loss of meaning in the nursing experience often precipitates the decision to leave the profession (Muldary 1983), whilst it could be argued that to be effective, nurses must be able to find meaning in their nursing practice.

Arnold (1989) suggests for nursing to be meaningful it would seem to require involvement, commitment and a sense of purpose. But if nurses lose these feelings, perhaps because the level of involvement becomes so intense it overrides their ability to cope, it seems likely to have a direct effect on the quality of care they are delivering. This is supported by Benner and Wrubel (1989) who refer to this loss of interest and enthusiasm and a sense of extreme fatigue as 'burnout' and state people in 'burnout' have literally lost the ability to care.

With so many frustrations and anxieties that nurses now face, it is argued that they may benefit from considering the meaning of their professional practice. This may help them in actively confronting difficulties and resolving conflicts rather than suppressing them. In so doing, they may foster an approach to their care that has possibly greater sensitivity and compassion.

By addressing their own meaning and purpose in life nurses may not completely work out their own belief system, as this often takes time and more life experiences. However they may feel 'less uncomfortable' in discussing such concerns with their patients.

Beliefs and convictions relating to mortality

Beliefs varied about peoples own mortality and involved a variety of issues, identified below.

Consideration of own mortality

Some nurses stated that they had not seriously considered their own mortality before. One offered an explanation for this:

> It's not something you want to think of really - you push it to the background.

However there were others who had given it some thought for different reasons:

> In college we were encouraged to consider our own mortality (!).

Another stated she had considered it because of a dependant and had consequently made her will and appropriate arrangements in the event of her death.

Life after death

This issue of what happened after death was raised by several nurses. One stated she would like to know if there was "another place" after death, whilst others admitted they were "curious" and "intrigued" as to what was beyond. Some explained that they did not know what there was but thought there could be "something". For them it was quite "reassuring" and "comforting." They could not give any further beliefs or explanation.

One nurse did however give her perceptions as to what happened after death:

I believe your body is like a box - if you like for your soul - and what you bury in the ground isn't the actual person, it's just the remainder, the shell of the person you actually knew... the soul is like the spirit and this leaves your body and goes onto better things and what is left is just the packaging.

The nature of death

Most nurses confessed they were not frightened by their own mortality, although one admitted that she wouldn't say it didn't worry her. Nevertheless for some there were anxieties concerning the "way" they might die:

I wouldn't want to suffer when I'm about to die.

I don't think I'm frightened of it... the only thing is I hope somebody can make sure I'm not in pain... I see death as inevitable but there is a quality to it.

For others there were fears for those who would be left behind eg. family:

I don't want to die before my child is old enough to look after himself- that is the only thing I am afraid of.

I don't mind dying for myself but for the people who would be grieving my loss. Mum and Dad have put so much into the family, it would hurt them so much if they outlived any one of us - the children.

It would seem that many of these thoughts about 'dying' are consistent with descriptions of feelings given by dying patients (McGilloway 1985b). Yet for most of these nurses, it was the first time they had actively considered their own mortality.

The importance of nurses analysing their own feelings and beliefs concerning death is strongly advocated by Winkelstein (1989). Although she discusses spirituality and the death of a child, her comments can be applied to the dying adult or one who is faced with the possibility of death. She considers such self examination is crucial, because the influence of nurses' ideas and beliefs will be felt either openly or more subtlety. If the main essence of nurse/patient interactions is the therapeutic use of self, then nurses will communicate their willingness to care, listen, accept and understand. Yet if nurses fail to recognise their own spiritual values and beliefs about human suffering and death, they may possibly be overcome by the sadness or horror of their patients' death and be unable to help or respond as they struggle to come to terms with their own beliefs and feelings. The development of such spiritual awareness appears essential in any educational programme concerning spirituality.

For the majority of the nurses religion was not of major significance in their lives. Some were quite categorical in their answers, "not at all", "nothing", "I don't use it at all", or during the interview stated "I'm not a religious person" or "I don't believe." Others were less clear. One felt she was "a bit confused about it" because she thought a lot of sightings of ghosts were valid:

I think there is a kind of supernatural something in existence - I just don't like the church.

Another admitted:

I wouldn't like to stand up and say there is absolutely nothing there, there is no God but it's not something I believe strongly and I don't derive any particular faith from it.

Nevertheless for two nurses religion was significant.

I wouldn't say it was top priority but I usually pray if I need something. I know I shouldn't, but I do.

Without religion things would get rather desperate at times and I have used God and prayer to get me through times when I have needed help. I enjoy going to church, the whole atmosphere and the singing and the prayer that gives me strength. I top up my need.

Definitions of God

All respondents attempted to describe God but with varying degrees of difficulty:

> *I don't know - I don't think I could put a sentence on it, because I don't really know what I believe.*

> *I don't know what God means, I haven't thought of that one.*

However with further open questioning, many began to clarify their thoughts and ideas. Some then found it easier to describe God in terms of who and what he was not.

> *I don't think that if there is a God it is a kind of thinking entity. I don't believe there's a man with a beard sitting there saying "you've done wrong - zapping with thunderbolt".*

> *I don't picture him as a lovely little man with a beard and white robe.*

Yet other descriptions were in terms of what God did or what God was for them. This seemed to depend on the strength of their religious beliefs. For those whose belief in God was strong, the descriptions were clear:

> *God is just a person, the overall, the maker, he is the overall who gives you choices in what life will hold for you and you have to make a choice and you either take the wrong choice or the right choice.*

> *He's aware of what's going on in the world, he's there all around - no gender but a spirit, a powerful spirit.*

> *God is love, somebody you go to if you need love and gives you a purpose in life - somebody to whom I pray and talk.*

Another considered 'God' to be a type of attitude or feeling:

> *To me God isn't a person; it's more of an attitude ... a humanistic attitude ... treating others as you hope they would treat you. It's*

general compassion, kindness, no cruelty. It's an overall feelings perhaps of warmth and compassion.

For the case study, religion was not a significant part of her life, although she appreciated its importance to other people. However she had clear ideas about who and what God was to her:

Religions are all stepping stones along the way and they all lead to the top of the mountain... God is like the top of the mountain, not that we would ever get to it. But the power is all pervading.

It seemed from these descriptions that for those nurses who had a strong sense of religion or who had actively considered their spirituality before, there was a much greater ability to articulate thoughts and beliefs, than for those who had not. In addition these nurses appeared to have fewer problems with questions relating to the meaning and purpose of life and suffering.

This is not to say that all nurses should base their beliefs on some kind of religious framework. Far from it. However coping with 'life' and indeed 'nursing' without firm, settled convictions and some kind of ideological framework, could lead to serious doubt and uncertainty.

Cluff (1986) notes that often patients, particularly those who are dying, question their beliefs, expose their religious concerns and wish to discuss their relationship with a 'Higher Being'. Yet they do not expect 'theological' answers from the listener who is often the nurse (Jacik 1989).

What seems more desirable is a 'comfortable listener'. Therefore if nurses attempt to address their own spiritual dimensions by examining the beliefs and principles which guide their own lives, they may feel more prepared to explore, with their patients, issues relating to the meaning of life, the battle with illness and the separation, loss and loneliness that they, the patients, may be facing.

Sources of love, hope and strength

As might be expected these sources varied for each individual nurse.

Relationships

For some, relationships with people were significant sources of love and hope.

"Friends", "work colleagues" and "generally people around you" were identified as sources of strength.

The family

But it was "the family" that was cited by most nurses as being the most significant source of love and hope and strength. Although many did not identify specific people, a few referred to particular family members eg. "parents," "spouses", "brothers/sisters", "their children."

Some gave an insight into their family relationships and background. One stated:

We're a very small, very close family... We keep in contact. I do get a lot of support from that and I certainly did years ago when I was leaving home because I always knew there was somebody there. I could strike out and if it failed it didn't matter but I could just go back and start again and that's very important - it's security... it would have been a close personal friendship when I was younger, the relationship I had with my parents, now it's the relationship I have with my husband. If anything should happen to him it would be unthinkable to me .... that's where I get my strength from.

For another, an important source of love was:

the way your family are with you and having a child... the fact my child is so dependent on me and you've got to be there for him. If you are loved then you can love other people.

The child's dependence on her made her realise how much he needed her.

Upbringing

Some nurses also identified their upbringing as providing love, hope and strength:

The way you have been treated when you were young and the way you have been brought up.

It stems from my upbringing. I've had a good religious upbringing and have a strong family background. So I've learnt to forgive, and trust in God and just take things from day to day, not being judgemental if I can help it and coming to terms with problems as they arise using my own intelligence.

Belief systems

For some nurses, religion was a significant source of love, hope and strength. One stated she found her religious beliefs comforting although she did not go to church on a regular basis:

I've got my own religious beliefs. I'm actually Catholic - I do go to Church - not on a regular basis any more but I do attend fairly regularly every Sunday. But I do believe there is a God and personally for me I think that's always comforting. Usually I do pray if I want something or am worried about something - it's someone to turn to.

Another stated her source of strength was partly religious although:

I do believe in certain things, but I just find it very hard to actually believe in it all.

For some other nurses their strength came from their belief that:

I just think it will always get better, whatever happens. I know that given time it will sort itself out.

I just know things will get better... if I'm particularly down, I'll cheer up eventually and forget about it.

The case study's sources also came from her belief system.

My belief in the universal power of love. Some people would call that God, some people would call it divinity. Whatever, there are all sorts of names for it, it doesn't really matter. To me it's not a personality... it is this all knowing power. You know it's something that is very humbling to recognise and know that life has a purpose - that's very important. For me it's a reason to be. It gives me purpose in life to know whatever one suffers it is all for a good cause in the end and to keep on keeping on.

Inner strength

Nevertheless some nurses recognised an inner strength:

I think I am a strong person.

I have a source of strength - it's in my nature.

Nursing

Yet for many of the nurses, nursing itself figured as a strong source of hope, love and strength.

It is not anything I believe in, it's what I see when I'm nursing...because you realise that life is all too short. It doesn't stop the arguing at home but it stops me walking out on an argument.

Meeting people, seeing people caring for each other and seeing everybody's Ok. Caring for patients, following their care through if they went to another ward if you had spent a lot of time with them.

For one nurse, nursing was the greatest source of love, hope and strength.

People I have met in my nursing career - patients; I have learnt so much from patients and how they are always so thankful for everything you do for them it's taught me to be humble... You put on a uniform and you immediately assume a sense of having strength. People rely on you and grasp strength from you. Yet when you see what some patients go through that gives you strength.

The values and beliefs elicited in these particular descriptions appear to emphasize the importance of relationships. As Stoll (1979) notes, relationships of trust and mutual understanding are one of the principle sources of hope, love and strength whether it be with family, friends or with a 'Higher Being.'

These were seen as the main resources that the individuals could draw upon in times of 'trouble' and 'despair' and as such could be referred to as 'external' sources. The sources occurring from 'within' the individual eg. inner strengths and belief systems could therefore be referred to as 'internal' sources.

In taking responsibility for themselves and their actions, nurses are often involved in facing up to problems and issues and dealing with them as best they can. They do this with the help of all their sources of love, hope and strength. Yet theories of motivation which attempt to explain the reasons why people behave in one way and not another, advocate the effectiveness of internal motivators such as the need for success and achievement, over and above external motivators such as rewards like encouragement or praise (Atkinson et al 1981). Thus it may be that internal sources of strength and support are more effective than external sources.

However whether they are internal or external, it may be that nurses need to clearly identify their own sources of strength and support in order to be able to deal with the issues and conflicts that arise in nursing practice. Furthermore, if there is lack of clarity as to where these sources come from, it may be that the coping mechanisms in dealing with such stresses cannot be activated.

Summary

It seems that for several reasons nurses may benefit from confronting their own spirituality. Not only will they possibly become more attuned to their patients' spiritual concerns but they may feel more at ease when these issues are raised. Furthermore it seems that having a clearer ideological framework of beliefs, be they non-religious or religious, the easier it may be to answer such questions about the meaning and purpose of life and reasons for suffering. This in turn may then help nurses cope with conflicts and issues that arise in their professional practise and in their own lives.

In any spirituality educational programme for nurse, it is necessary for them to be given the opportunity to consider their own personal beliefs and become more aware of their own spiritual dimension.

Furthermore, in highlighting these issues, nurses' belief systems appear to have an important influence on nursing actions and interventions and subsequently on their interactions with their patients.

7 Educational issues

Although modified aspects of a grounded theory approach have been used in this study, it must be noted that this is not a true grounded theory study. Whilst there is little research about the topic under consideration, spirituality has been described and discussed in some detail in the literature. Therefore the research was not addressing something 'new'. Grounded theory however, is usually used to explore an unknown field.

Furthermore, constant comparative analysis advocated by Glaser and Strauss (1967) was not used. This is where each interview transcript is compared with the previous one, in order to modify and amend future interviews. In this study the aim was to explore nurses' perceptions of spirituality in order to highlight their understanding of the concept, not to develop complex explanations of relationships.

Nevertheless, what did emerge from the study was that nurses' personal beliefs could have an influence, not only on their nursing actions, but on nurse/patient interactions. Whilst this could be tentatively described as a model/framework for nursing practice, it is felt that further research should be undertaken to explore these issues.

A great deal of information was obtained from the rich descriptions given by the trained nurses and the case study. In view of the quantity of this qualitative data, it may have been more realistic to only consider one aspect of the trained nurses' perceptions, either personal spirituality or related to their professional practice. Nevertheless, this approach may not have identified the suggestion that there is a relationship between nurses' personal beliefs and their nursing practice or indeed the need for further research into these issues.

Certainly no generalisations can be drawn from this study. Yet a great deal has been learnt and there have been a number of consequences. The researcher has now led many sessions on spirituality and nursing practice for both pre and post-registration students. As a result much discussion has been generated amongst the nurses.

Several students commented that they found the sessions 'very moving' and had raised issues for them that had not been addressed before. One group of post-basic students have subsequently formed a 'spiritual awareness' group, inviting outside speakers to come and talk and facilitate discussions about different belief systems.

In teaching such sessions, the researcher has become acutely aware of the personal nature of such a topic and the many emotions that it may evoke. Indeed some people, other than the interviewees, who have been involved with the study (family, friends, colleagues), have spontaneously expressed how different thoughts and emotions have arisen as a result of thinking about or reading the study. Such emotions are of relevance, not only when dealing with the spiritual dimensions of nurses but also when dealing with the spiritual dimensions of patients.

Indeed once the study was completed, it stimulated much thought and informal discussion amongst the clinical staff who had been involved with the project. Whilst none had been at all 'distressed' by the interviews, many felt they had been' enlightened'. It may have been beneficial to have reinterviewed these nurses to establish in more detail their reactions to considering such issues.

Overall this study has attempted to provide a greater understanding about the concept of spirituality. However it strongly urges further studies relating to spirituality and nursing practice.

Other issues arising out of the findings

There seemed to be a central paradox arising out of some of the interviewees' responses: spiritual beliefs are often thought to be 'personal' and yet the notion of God and of spiritual belief is often thought to be universal. How can such an apparent paradox be resolved? How does it impinge of the care of patients? If, on the one hand, nurses should not bring their personal beliefs to bear on the care of their patients, how should they act? If they are asked, outright, about their religious beliefs, are they duty bound a) to tell the truth and b) to share their own views?

If spiritual issues should be discussed in training programmes for nurses, at what point should these ideas be introduced? If one takes the view that the spiritual is an integral part of all persons and that nurses should care for the whole person, then it follows that such issues should be discussed from early in a training course. On the other hand, if spiritual issues are also 'personal' ones, do nurse teachers have the right to discuss such personal issues and to expect students to *want* to discuss such issues?

Can there be 'training' in this area? What form would such training take? Would it involve, simply, a relatively neutral exploration of each person's beliefs, with no final conclusion being drawn from such a discussion? Would it involve a form of comparative religious training with inputs from Christians, Muslims, Hindus, atheists and so forth? Or would it involve some sort of training in pastoral counselling with nurses being helped to explore patients' spiritual problems and helping them to find answers?

Who might undertake to teach any sort of spiritual training programme for student nurses? Should *all* nurse teachers have a hand in such a programme or should the topic be taught be a subject specialist? What sort of background would be appropriate for such a specialist: would they, for example, be expected to have a Bachelor of Divinity degree? If all teachers where expected to address spiritual issues, what could or should be done about the teacher who was 'spiritually neutral' and felt that spiritual issues were not particular important?

Conclusions and recommendations

From this small, qualitative study of nurses' perceptions of spirituality it would appear that further clarification of the notion of spirituality both personally and in terms of professional practice is required by nurses who practice clinical and by those who teach the topic. Although some nurses use some of the essential components of spiritual care, it is not comprehensively addressed in clinical practice. Furthermore analysis of the data suggests that the nurses' own belief systems have some affect on their nursing actions and nurse/patient interactions. This tentative model/framework for practice requires further development. From the study, it would appear that a nurse's personal belief system impinges on her nursing actions (particularly when the context is spirituality). It would seem that nurses who have no particular training in the field are thrown back on their own beliefs. When these are 'religious' in nature, some nurses will use those religious beliefs to guide them in the discussions with patients. The effect of these nursing actions seems likely to effect the nurse/patient relationship, generally and this may or may not bring changes in the personal belief system of the nurse. Similarly, the *outcome* of a nurse/patient relationship may also effect the nurse's belief system. Nurses, like all most other people, do not live in isolation. They are affected by the people they meet and by the things that happen to them. As we have seen, many nurses have, regularly, to face traumatic and life-threatening situations - often as observers. It seems likely that these observations and subsequent reflection on them is, again, likely to affect the nurse's belief system.

It is suggested, therefore, that at least three areas need to be considered when helping to prepare nurses for work in the spiritual domain: the nurse's personal belief system, the actions they carry out as a nurse and the nurse/patient relationship. Each, as we have seen, is related to the other.

Nurses may well benefit from not only examining in more detail this concept in relation to nursing practice but also in relation to their own personal beliefs.

This has obvious implications for nurse education and this chapter offers some suggestions as to the ways in which nurses could be better prepared for their role as spiritual carers.

The curriculum

This study has identified the complexity of the concept of spirituality and its relationship to ethics, morals, culture, religion and self awareness. A curriculum that incorporates these themes would allow a more integrated approach to spiritual issues. This in turn may help nurses consider spirituality as an integral part of care, not something 'special' or only appropriate for certain groups of patients.

Spirituality workshops

The use of study days given over to spiritual aspects of care is advocated, the aims being to explore the notion of spirituality as applied to nurses themselves and to patient care. In view of the range of issues that need addressing, it is suggested that several study days would be required rather than attempting to cover all aspects in one day.

Group work is suggested as an appropriate 'education method' as this would allow the students to learn from each other and benefit from each others' ideas. However to allow free participation and discussion, the group size should be restricted to 6-8 students. It is vitally important that students feel relaxed and unthreatened and it is necessary to point out that although they are invited to actively participate, they should feel under no obligation to do so. An introduction which includes setting clear ground rules at the beginning of such workshops/study days would enable this point to be emphasized. This would also allow the reinforcement of such issues as maintaining confidentiality, respecting each other as individuals and valuing each others opinions.

Seating arrangements are also very important and an informal, closed circle may facilitate debate and reduce any 'psychological distance' between members of the group and the facilitator or group leader. The content of learning could be divided into three sections:

- Exploring the nurses' own spiritual dimensions whereby they could reflect on their own beliefs and values and sources of love, hope and strength, with another person and then feedback in a larger plenary session.
- Exploring other ideas and theories so giving some theoretical input using a multicultural approach. This could include non-religious and religious views.
- Application of the above discussion to nursing practice, covering such topics as relevance to nursing practice, the essential skills for spiritual assessment and spiritual care. Experiential learning could be used to develop nurses' communication and counselling skills and enhance their therapeutic use of self, as well as introducing complementary approaches to medicine.

These sessions should be concluded with some kind of evaluation that would allow the nurses to consider what they had learnt from the workshops.

Experiential learning

It has been suggested, above, that the experiential learning approach to learning might be a useful approach to exploring spirituality with nurses and with nursing students. Experiential learning methods are ones that call, directly, on students' own life and work experiences. Through a process of reflection on experience and group discussion, students learn not only to develop their own beliefs and ideas but become tolerant of others' views. Such an approach to learning is based on the notion of 'andragogy' or the theory and practice of the education of adults. The American educator, Malcolm Knowles, has used the term 'andragogy' to describe negotiated adult learning as opposed to 'pedagogy' or teacher-directed, child education (Knowles 1980). Knowles argues that negotiated and experiential learning those types of education best suited to adults because:

- Adults both desire and enact a tendency toward self-directednes as they mature, though they may be dependent in certain situations.
- Adults' experiences are a rich resource for learning. Adults learn more effectively though experiential techniques of education such as discussion or problem-solving.
- Adults are aware of specific learning needs generated by real life tasks or problems. Adult education programs, therefore, should be organised around 'life application' categories and sequenced according to learners' readiness to learn.
- Adults are competency based learners in that they wish to apply newly acquired skills or knowledge to their immediate circumstances. Adults are, therefore, 'performance centred' in their orientation to learning. (Knowles 1980).

All of these aspects of adult learning are appropriate in the teaching and learning of nursing and in the discussion of spiritual issues. All learners coming to nurse education do so as adults. Whatever criteria are used to measure adulthood, it would be difficult to argue otherwise. They all bring to the learning situation a wealth of personal and occupational experience: no learners in nursing arrive as *tabula rasa* or 'blank slates'. All nurses, too, need to use the skills they learn for practical purposes within their lives and within their jobs. So, too, do they need to apply what they learn in practical settings. All of these aspects of adult learning are also consonant with the learning approaches, described throughout this book, in that they emphasise the use of a balance between knowledge, practice and personal experience as the keystones of learning nursing.

Knowles and associates (1984) have identified seven components of andragogical practice that they feel are replicable in a variety of programmes and training workshops throughout the world. These components are highly relevant to the development of nursing skills and nursing knowledge:

- Facilitators must establish a physical and psychological climate conducive to learning. This is achieved physically by circular seating arrangements and psychologically by creating a climate of mutual respect among all participants, by emphasising collaborative modes of learning, by establishing an atmosphere of mutual trust, by offering to be supportive and by emphasising that learning is pleasant.
- Facilitators must involve learners in mutual planning of methods and curriculum directions. People will make firm commitments to activities which they feel they have played a participatory, contributory role.
- Facilitators must involve themselves in diagnosing their own learning needs.
- Facilitators must encourage learners to formulate their own learning objectives.
- Facilitators must encourage learners to identify resources and to devise strategies for using such resources to accomplish their objectives.
- Facilitators must help learners to carry out their learning plans.
- Facilitators must involve learners in evaluating their learning, principally through the use of qualitative evaluation modes.

Out of this discussion on the philosophical underpinnings of two approaches to the curriculum arise certain practical considerations for programme planing for nurses training in the domain of spiritual matters. Brookfield (1986) discusses what he calls the principles of practice in community action projects. These principles may well serve as the underlying principles for developing curricula for the training and education of nurses:

- The medium of learning and action is the small group.
- Essential to the success of efforts is the development of collaborative solidarity among group members. This does not mean that dissension is silenced or divergence stifled; rather, group members are able to accept conflict, secure in the knowledge that their peers regard their continued presence in the group as vital to its success.

- The focus of the group's actions is determined after full discussion of participant's needs and full negotiation of all needs, including those of any formal 'educators' present.
- As adults undertake the actions they have collaboratively agreed upon, they develop an awareness of their collective power. This awareness is also felt when these adults renegotiate aspects of their personal, occupational and recreational lives.
- A successful initiative is one in which action and analysis alternate. Concentrating solely on action allows no time for the group to check its progress or alter previously agreed-upon objectives. But if the members of the group engage solely in analysis, they will never come to recognize their individuality and collective power. Empowerment is impossible without alternating action and reflection. (Brookfield 1986).

If Knowles and Brookfield are right, adults need to use what they learn. All learning about nursing (and, perhaps, especially in the spiritual domain) needs to be grounded in the participants practical experience and any new learning needs to be the sort that can be applied on future occasions. Both Knowles' and Brookfields' notions of the educational principles of facilitating learning groups are entirely relevant to the running of learning groups for nurses in that all learners coming to such groups (regardless of their status and regardless of the specific discipline) are adults. All of these principles apply to the exploration of spiritual issues with nurses. As we have suggested, there is likely to be little place in such education or training for prescription or dogma and most nurse educators are likely to need to use an andragogical or experiential approach to teaching and learning in this delicate area.

Experiential learning has received considerable coverage in the recent literature on nurse education (Raichura 1987, Tomlinson, 1985, Kagan, Evans and Kay 1986, Miles 1987). The theoretical literature seems to use the term in two different ways. One approach involves the concept of life as a learning process and thus experiential learning is learning through the process of living, working and generally relating to the world. This approach to the concept of experiential learning is best exemplified by Keeton and his associates (1976).

The other approach is via humanistic psychology and emphasises subjective experience, personal interpretation and the education of the emotions. This approach is best exemplified in the writings of Kilty (1983), Shaffer (1978) and Heron (1973, 1982, 1977).

One of the problems with Heron's work is that it is insufficiently referenced and thus it is difficult to place his work in context. He seems to draw from a wide variety of sources, including encounter, gestalt and humanistic psychology. He has recently made his interest in mysticism and transpersonal psychology more overt (1987). Through the Human Potential Research Project at the University of Surrey, he has had much to do with influencing the ways in which nurse lecturers have adopted the experiential learning approach to nurse education. He has also explored, in some detail, the 'transpersonal' domain of psychology: that which is concerned with metaphysical and spiritual aspects.

Apart from these two main themes in the experiential learning literature, there are also some 'hybrids'. Kolb (1984), for example, combines some of the 'learning through the process of living' approach with ideas from Carl Rogers and Carl Jung and applies, almost paradoxically, a fairly rigorous quantitative approach to researching his theoretical constructs. Boydel's (1976) theoretical approach also seems to stand outside the mainstream humanistic approach and yet does not fit completely into the first approach either.

Experiential knowledge

One of the present writers has proposed the idea of experiential learning being defined through a theory of knowledge (1987). Three types of knowledge have been proposed: propositional, practical and experiential knowledge. Propositional knowledge is 'textbook' knowledge of facts, theories and models. Practical knowledge is knowledge revealed through practice-for example the demonstration of successfully giving an injection or the demonstration of effective counselling skills. Experiential knowledge is personal knowledge, gained through direct encounter with a person, place or thing. It is that knowledge that we 'know' for ourselves and that cannot easily be transmitted to other people. Experiential learning, then, is any learning which increases the facilitation of experiential knowledge. In this way, it is differentiated from traditional learning methods which, arguably, have mostly been concerned with the development of propositional or practical knowledge. The domain of experiential knowledge may be bound up with the notion of spirituality. Arguably, we only 'know' what we know about the spiritual domain through this personal and idiosyncratic approach.

Nursing lecturers' views of experiential learning

This, then, is a brief overview of the literature. Nurse lecturers, it would seem are less certain about how to define experiential learning. In research into the field, it is emerging that nurse educators interpret the concept of experiential learning in widely differing ways (Burnard 1989). Some, for instance, see it only as a means of teaching certain topics, notably interpersonal skills. Others see it as applicable to all nursing topics including law and anatomy and physiology. Some see the approach as being concerned with learning from practical experience (including clinical placements) whilst others see it as more concerned with 'personal' learning and self awareness. Yet others view experiential learning as being concerned mainly with role play and compare and contrast it to more 'traditional' methods such as the lecture. Some are fairly zealous in their adoption of experiential learning and base their entire curriculum on in it, whilst others see it as one of a range of teaching methods.

Both the literature and the lecturers that the present writer has talked to are in agreement on two issues: that experiential learning is concerned with personal experience and with 'practice' rather than theory. Sometimes those issues are overlaid with fairly complicated theories about the person- often humanistic or transpersonal. In other cases, the approach is essentially pragmatic: the process of learning by doing is a practical aid to developing certain skills.

In passing, it is interesting to reflect on why the humanistic and transpersonal themes have emerged in nurse education at this time, given that they developed and perhaps reached a peak in the 1960's. Much of the 'classic' humanistic theory was worked out in the 60's (Jourard 1964, Rogers 1967, Roszak 1969). Humanistic psychology has had little impact on traditional academic psychology, as the late Carl Rogers noted recently (1985), and the encounter movement is certainly less pervasive than it used to be.

At least two, very speculative, reasons for the current interest in the humanistic approach to experiential learning in nurse education can be mooted. One concerns the age of nurse lecturers. Because of the career path leading to the post of nurse lecturer, many lecturers will be of an age where they can recall the 60's and may have 'brought with them' the attitudes and values of that period. The second, is the publication of the 1982 syllabus of training for psychiatric nursing students (ENB 1982). This syllabus was formulated, to some degree, by people who had a considerable interest in humanistic psychology. Many aspects of the syllabus reflect the humanistic approach and the syllabus has been influential in aspects of nurse education beyond psychiatric nursing. The syllabus is also unusual in that it recommends that experiential learning methods be used.

Andragogy

Andragogy, a term associated with Malcolm Knowles (Knowles 1978, Knowles 1980, Knowles 1984), though used before his time, is one used to differentiate the theory and practice of adult education from pedagogy- the theory and practice of the education of children. Knowles claimed that adults differed in some fundamental ways from children and, therefore, required a different educational system.

Out of these ideas, Knowles drew up a method of conducting adult education sessions. One objection that may be raised about Knowles' theory is that the ideas identified above may be applicable, also, to children. If this is the case, it is difficult to see how he can argue for a discreet theory of adult education based on these principles. Knowles acknowledges this problem and, in later writing, tends to describe andragogy as an attitude towards education rather than as being a discreet theory of adult education. This argument and others relating to andragogy have been well described by Jarvis (1983, 1984) and Brookfield (1987).

Andragogy has much in common with the student-centred learning approach of the late Carl Rogers (1984). This is not surprising as both Knowles and Rogers were influenced, through their respective professors of education, by John Dewey, the pragmatist and philosopher of education (Dewey 1966, 1971, Kirschenbaum 1979). It also has much in common with many of the approaches to experiential learning, emphasising, as they do, the centrality of personal experience and subjective interpretation.

Another observation that may be made about both andragogy and experiential learning is that they are both very American in their approach. The American educational system, influenced as it has been by Dewey's work, has always tended towards a more student-centred, individualistic approach to education. It was something of a surprise, therefore, for one of the present writers to find little or no evidence of experiential learning methods being regularly used in the parts of California, Florida and New England, visited early in 1987 (Burnard 1987). The accent, there, was very much on learning to pre-set, prescribed objectives. In California, particularly, 'experiential learning' was something associated with the encounter movement of the 1960's. On the east coast, and particularly around New York, humanistic psychology was often not recognised as a separate school of psychology at all. Whether or not all this means that we are behind or ahead of the Americans in terms of modern approaches to nurse education, is a moot point. Some would argue that we have arrived at student centred learning rather late in the day. Others would no doubt argue that we are putting into practice what American educators have been preaching for years.

Application

How, then, may aspects of experiential learning and andragogy usefully be combined in nurse education and, in particular, in the spiritual domain? Such a combination needs to take into account certain basic principles such as negotiation, the importance of personal experience and the use of self and peer assessment. What must also be born in mind, however, is that learner nurses and nurse lecturers have to work to a prescribed syllabus of training laid down by the English and Welsh National Boards. This fact makes nurse education somewhat different to many of the experiential learning training workshops at which all of the content may arise out of participants needs and wants. Many nurse lecturers may encounter problems in translating workshop experience into practice because of this fact. Also, there is a large difference between using experiential learning methods in a two-day to one-week training workshop and using them on a regular basis throughout a three year programme.

A three stage model may be described. In stage one, two things happen. First, the students identify their own learning needs through direction from the lecturer and in line with the 'learning contract' approach described by Knowles (1975). Second, the lecturer identifies certain learning needs out of the prescribed syllabus. The students can draw from their previous ward experience, here, and may find a 'brainstorming' session a useful means of generating topics.

Thus, in stage two, a timetable is negotiated. It will consist of the two elements described above and may be divided into a 'theory' element and a 'skills' element. The skills element may include both practical nursing skills and interpersonal skills, as appropriate. Again, it will be remembered that the content of this theory and skills mix will arise jointly out of the expressed needs of the students and the suggested ideas of the nurse lecturer.

The theory element may then be learned using a whole range of educational approaches, including the traditional ones of lecture and seminar, as required. However, for the skills element, it is recommended that the experiential learning cycle be followed. All of this seems particular appropriate for the teaching and learning of such a 'delicate' topic as spiritual care. Whilst lectures on the topic no doubt have their place, it would seem more appropriate that lecturers encourage students to reflect on their own beliefs and values and to examine who they might talk to patients about spirituality. The experiential approach seems ideal for this sort of work.

Self and peer evaluation

Following the learning of both theory and practice, learners are called upon to self and peer evaluate their new learning. Again, this has been described elsewhere (Burnard 1987, Kilty 1978). Essentially, the aim is to encourage learner autonomy by developing in those learners the ability to check the learning development of themselves and their colleagues. At this stage, too, it is usually necessary (if not mandatory) to include the more 'objective' evaluation processes that are instigated by lecturers: examinations, tests, questionnaires, check lists and so forth. Out of this evaluation phase can emerge and evolve a new assessment phase and thus the cycle continues.

Student-centred learning

The cycle, briefly outlined here incorporates the student-centred, negotiating approach of andragogy with the accent on personal experience and self and peer evaluation of experiential learning. It also acknowledges that learner nurses need to work to a syllabus and that nurse lecturers can contribute much to effectively planning a course of study around such a syllabus. In this cycle, 'negotiation' means just that- the programme emerges out of the experience and knowledge of both students and lecturers. In recent years it has been almost as if lecturers where required to remain quietly in the background and ensure that they never inflicted their views on their learners! Whilst it would be difficult to sensibly advocate a return to the days of a totally prescribed course of training, it seems reasonable to acknowledge the educational skill of lecturers in helping students to build an effective programme of nursing education.

Perhaps, then, it is a question of developing a balance between what Heron

(1986) calls 'following' and 'leading'. Following involves taking the lead from the students, using their experience and ideas. Leading, on the other hand, means making suggestions and using structure to help the students. Together, these methods can ensure balance and symmetry in the nurse education programme. If the programme involves too much 'following' or is too student-directed in its methods, it will be unbalanced. On the other hand, if it involves too much 'leading' or is too teacher-directed in its methods, it will also be unbalanced.

Having said this, the attitude towards nurse education should always remain student centred. The issue is not whether or not the lecturer or the student should serve as the focal point of the educational process but the means by which the students educational needs are identified and satisfied. In this sense, then, the focus remains the student. Again, given the idiosyncratic nature of many people's belief systems, it would seem appropriate that the student-centred approach be adopted by nurse educators who are planning to explore the spiritual domain with their students.

Objections

There may, of course, be some practical objections to this combined approach. First, the approach takes time. it is far easier and less time consuming if the lecturer prepares the timetable and the lessons. However, the negotiated approach is likely to yield a more appropriate timetable, geared to this group of students, at this time.

Second, it is likely that many students have been socialised into a more teacher-directed and teacher-centred approach. In the present writer's experience it takes time for such students to adapt to the approach suggested here but when they do, they seem to prefer it to the more traditional approach. Some, of course, do not prefer it and it seems reasonable to take into account the needs and wants of the other-directed student. Not everyone, after all, is necessarily self-directed (Reisman 1950).

Third, there is the question of 'getting through the syllabus'. This seems a sensible issue to consider as, like it or not, students have to sit examinations during and at the end of their training. Whilst the literature on the question of content in the curriculum offers various views of what should, could or may be included in a nurse training course (Cork 1987, Greaves 1987, Beattie 1987), in the end, all schools of nursing are constrained, at least to some degree, by syllabuses prescribed by the National Boards (this may, of course, change with the introduction of the recommendations of Project 2000). If the negotiated approach, as indicated here, is used and the syllabus is repeatedly referred back to as a sourcebook for guidance, then such problems should not arise. The accent, here, is on negotiation: the lecturer should be free to recommend that certain aspects of the syllabus be introduced at certain stages of training. As we noted above, the student-centred approach to education should never mean that the lecturer is redundant in the educational process and she should feel free to exercise judgement in such aspects of curriculum planning. In the end, however, no course of training, traditional or negotiated, ever covers every aspect of the syllabus.

Other considerations

Even if nurses' understanding of spirituality is increased through better education, it does not guarantee that patients' spiritual needs will be addressed or met. Clinical areas need to be adequately staffed to allow nurses to spend the necessary time with patients. There needs to be the adoption of a system of care that facilitates the development of a trusting, empathetic nurse/patient relationship such as primary nursing or the very least, patient allocation. Furthermore it is suggested that an explicit theory/model of nursing would help guide a systematic approach to organising nursing care. Finally, it would seem that nurses have spiritual dimensions that require consideration. Counselling or peer support groups may enable nurses to discuss their feelings in a supportive atmosphere and may provide a regular opportunity to talk through their problems and stresses, so developing some form of effective coping mechanism. If patients' spiritual needs are to be met, it is vital that nurses care for themselves.

A personal experience of teaching

This study has offered an exploration of some concepts of spirituality as they apply to nursing. In the final section, the application of some of these ideas to practice is explored via the commentary of one of the researchers (JH). The commentary relates to the researcher's own experience of exploring the notion of spirituality with student nurses.

As a Nurse Tutor for Registered General Nurse Courses (last course completed January 1993) and Diploma in Nursing Studies Courses (Project

2000) with a particular interest in this aspect of care over the last 12 months, I have run a number of spirituality workshops.

This personal account of my experiences will cover such issues as:- the types of courses, the facilitators role, the teaching methods adopted, the preparation of other facilitators; spirituality; formal incorporation into nursing curriculum.

The facilitator's role

As already discussed, such workshops or study days should not be an exercise in proselytising. For this reason they should be led by a facilitator rather than a 'teacher' who has previously considered his/her own beliefs and who feels 'comfortable' in dealing with such issues and in discussing such aspects of life that have no specific answers or provable certainties.

The aim should be to explore and examine the notion of spirituality as it applies to nursing practice. This should be in an understanding and supportive atmosphere. Thus the facilitator needs to be skilled in ensuring the group is not dismissive of anyones ideas and can competently deal with any emotion as it arises.

Like Burnard (1988) I too find the process of facilitating such discussions both humbling and nerve racking. Humbling because they illuminate other peoples traumas and difficulties and so highlight my own insecurities and failings and nerve racking because I am never quite sure what personal issues are going to be raised or what 'can of worms' will be opened.

Nevertheless they are always interesting and most enlightening and it never ceases to amaze me that once the session has finished I am left not only with a feeling of exhilaration but also exhaustion.

Courses

Spirituality has been highlighted as an important dimension of individuals. Therefore as such, spiritual needs should not be confined to particular groups of patients/client, for example, the dying. For this reason, it is important that such sessions should be held for students on a variety of courses both pre-registration and post-basic.

In my experience, examples of courses that have included spirituality sessions have been: Registered General Nurse courses, common foundation programmes (Diploma in Nursing Studies), adult branches, child branches, mental health branches, ENB 237 and 240 adult and paediatric oncology courses, ENB 254 cardiac nursing courses, ENB 934 HIV/AIDS courses and courses at the local hospice.

At first as one of the co-ordinators for the high dependency/specialist terms for the Adult Branch of the Diploma in Nursing Studies Course, I was somewhat dubious at discussing nursing situations outside my realm of clinical experience and practice particularly concerning the child, mental health and oncology. But in preparation for such sessions I consequently broadened my reading and liaised closely with my branch and post-basic colleagues, so extending my own knowledge.

At the outset I am always honest about my background and having initially discussed the concept of spirituality, spiritual needs, spiritual health and spiritual distress, I have then 'thrown it over' to the particular group to draw their own conclusions as to its relevance to practice and how spiritual assessment and spiritual care can be realistically applied to their specialism.

This has appeared to be effective on two counts. Firstly the students have appreciated airing their own ideas and experiences drawing on their personal encounters with patients/clients. Secondly as someone with limited experience in their field, I have been able to contribute a different perspective to the debate. This has often been enlightening as well as amusing, but the session has always been conducted in a supportive atmosphere where the exchange of ideas and debate about nursing has been enhanced.

Content and teaching/learning methods

The content of such sessions has varied according to the amount of time allocated. But 2 hours has been enough time to cover:

- The concept of spirituality i.e. definitions of spirituality, spiritual needs, spiritual health, spiritual distress.
- An examination of the students' own spiritual needs.
- The relevance of spirituality to clinical practice.
  Follow up discussions at a later date also lasting 2 hours (approx) have included:
- Spiritual assessment in practice.
- spiritual care.

Only once have I attempted to address these issues by using a formal lecture to a large group of 45 students. However I would not advocate this type of teaching method for such a complex topic. In this situation students were the passive recipients of information and were unable to question and debate the points in order to gain some kind of appreciation of spirituality and its complexity.

Thus to date, the main teaching and learning method adopted has been group discussion, incorporating paired activities, brain storming, and evaluation exercises. The group sizes have ranged from 8-20.

At the outset I have found it useful to give some kind of introduction to myself, my nursing background and to clearly establish that my interest in spirituality has developed not from any particular religious perspective but from my own personal quest to understand this concept. This occurred during a taught Masters of Nursing Course when I had to submit an academic essay about meeting patients' spiritual needs in clinical practice.

These reasons and giving an overview of the aims and content of the session have appeared to go some way in overcoming the reluctance on the part of some students, about attending and participating in such a discussion.

Following this I have always negotiated with the participants, some ground rules. These have included confidentiality, valuing and respecting beliefs and ideas of others, being supportive to one another and the right to remain silent.

In most instances the group have known each other very well and have already set ground rules with their personal tutor. However, in most cases I have not met them before and so consider myself in their eyes to be somewhat of an unknown quantity. In my experience many private and personal thoughts, feelings and experiences have been raised and aired during the discussion. It is therefore essential that they feel the environment is safe and supportive enough to be able to share these thoughts and emotions without any fear of reprisal, recrimination or humiliation.

Often the issue of confidentiality needs clarification. In my opinion it alludes to not discussing, outside the confines of the room, any kind of personal detail/ experience or any client/ patient data that may be divulged by the group members. However, in order for students to increase their awareness and understanding of this notion, it may be that the general concept of spirituality, itself, needs debating beyond the classroom. The students, on the other hand, may have different ideas. Therefore I have found it worthwhile spending a few minutes exploring what they mean by the term 'confidentiality' and how it is to be applied to the session.

As someone who considers herself to be a 'quiet' member of discussion groups, more of a listener, I also consider the ground rule about the right to remain silent to be important. In my experience, during any discussion, there is nothing worse than feeling you are being pressurised or put on the spot to say something. Sometimes silence is needed in order to assimilate and mull over what has been said and it may be some time before thoughts and feelings can be expressed in words. This is particularly true when dealing with such a complex issue as spirituality.

Whilst this ground rule has always been included, it often crosses my mind as to whether this will put paid to any kind of debate whatsoever! However, on most occasions, it has been enthusiastically incorporated into the ground rules and so far I have never experienced a completely silent group.

On the whole students seem to have found difficulty in defining the term spirituality and have had to be coaxed to share their thoughts. With smaller groups (6-12) discussion has been easier to facilitate but with larger groups (12-20) I have found it helpful to divide the students into smaller groups of 5-6 or even pairs returning to the larger group for a plenary session at a later stage, once they feel more 'comfortable' with the topic. As the discussion has progressed I have contributed my own thoughts and ideas with references to the appropriate literature.

The degree to which I share my own personal experiences and feelings depends upon the group, the level of debate and on my own psychological state at the time. There have been times when I have considered that sharing my own experiences and feelings will help initiate discussion or even enhance the debate. But this sharing is always done consciously, bearing in mind that my role is that of facilitator. Such experiences are given in very general terms. For example, highlighting my own spiritual needs or giving instances when I have questioned the meaning of life. On the whole, this seems to have provided the students with ideas from which they can begin to think of their own spirituality. In addition, sharing part of myself appears to help foster a supportive, trusting atmosphere.

In my experience the students seem to appreciate the opportunity to air their feelings and ideas without feeling they have to 'take notes'. Of course the extent to which this applies varies from student to student but for those who wish to formalise their thoughts, each session has been accompanied by a reference list and has included those authors referred to and highlighted in the discussion.

It is always difficult to judge the effectiveness of any session but I have found it helpful to conclude with an evaluation exercise where each students has been asked to state one aspect they have enjoyed and least enjoyed about the session.

Many have expressed their surprise at having enjoyed the debate particularly since their expectations of such a lesson were often low. In addition many have commented that it has been the first time they have actively considered their own spirituality.

Yet more often than not they have stated that they have ben given 'food for thought' and wish to 'reflect' on the issues in their own time. I have always felt heartened by these responses since possibly all I can aim for in the initial session is to stimulate some spiritual awareness which could be built upon at a later date. I too have included myself in this final exercise. It never ceases to amaze me just how much some students are willing to divulge about themselves and their experiences.

Formal incorporation into nursing curriculum

As yet spirituality has not been formally written into the nursing curriculum of the Diploma in Nursing Studies Course. However, recently, during the latter part of the Common Foundation Programme, $2\frac{1}{2}$-3 hours was allocated to explore the issue of spirituality and the spiritual health of nurses. This was part of a 3 day workshop for the Diploma students entitled 'Caring for the Carers'.

These sessions not only addressed the notion of spirituality but also the spirituality of the nurses themselves and its relevance to nursing practice. It was envisaged that further sessions would follow once the students had commenced their Branch Programmes. They would then be better able to consider the feasibility of spiritual assessment and the components of spiritual care and so establish how spirituality could be realistically incorporated into clinical practice for a variety of client groups.

Certainly it does seem that as more spirituality sessions are being conducted so there is greater awareness about spirituality and nursing practice amongst the teaching staff. This, plus the formal incorporation of such topics as ethics, self awareness and sociological aspects of religion into the nursing curriculum, has been a positive move towards the integration of spirituality into a nurse education programme.

Preparation of other facilitators

The number of students within the Common Foundation Programme is 160 and this has necessitated preparing other teachers for facilitating these sessions. I approached 9 teachers with a variety of clinical backgrounds and included at least one from each Branch programme. In addition they were all experienced in conducting such philosophical debates and dealing with emotional issues that might arise. Furthermore they were people who, in my opinion, would not tackle the topic from any kind of strong religious perspective.

Prior to the session I gave each tutor a preparation pack which included a selection of reading material and reference list. I also held an informal discussion, so that we could share our concerns, anxieties and clarify any queries. Whilst I did not want to be prescriptive I also set out a suggested outline for the 3 hour session so we would roughly cover the same points.

This seemed to be appreciated and whilst each group varied it provided some kind of formal structure upon which the facilitators could base the discussion. At the end of the mornings session I spoke to each facilitator individually. This was primarily to obtain some kind of evaluation of the discussions. However, I began to realise that as facilitators we all needed to unwind and be 'debriefed'. Without exception we all felt the sessions had been worthwhile and stimulating but felt somewhat exhausted by the intensity of the debate and complexity of the topic. Nevertheless the majority of facilitators expressed an interest in being involved again, and indeed some have led such discussion groups since.

Sample activities for use in spirituality workshops

The previous sections have identified a number of approaches to 'teaching' the concept of spirituality to nursing students. It has been noted that the term 'facilitation' is probably a more appropriate one in this domain: the concept of spirituality appears to be too personal a one for didactic teaching to be appropriate. In this final section, some exercises for use in spirituality workshops are offered, based on the authors' experience of working with student groups. Many activities can be improvised but the following may give the potential facilitator some ideas about how to structure activities.

Activity 1

Aim of the activity

To explore participants views of spirituality.

Environmental requirements

A circle of chairs in a large room in which participants can pair off for the activity. Alternatively, a series of small rooms can be used for the pairs work and the group can reconvene in the larger.

Number in group

Between 5 and 20 participants

Process

The larger group pairs off. Each pair nominates one of them as A and the other as B. A asks of B, the question: 'What do you understand by the term spirituality?' and listens to the response. A answers the question as completely as possible until he or she has exhausted the topic. Then A and B switch roles and B asks the question of A and listens to the answer.

When all pairs have worked through the activity, the larger group reconvenes and the group facilitator encourages feedback and discussion of the answers to the question.

Evaluation activity

Each person, in turn, in the larger group is invited to say what they found most and least useful about the activity.

Activity 2

Aim of the activity

To explore the religious views of the group.

Environmental requirements

A circle of chairs in a large room in which participants can pair off for the activity. Alternatively, a series of small rooms can be used for the pairs work and the group can reconvene in the larger.

Number in group

Between 5 and 20 participants

Process

The group pairs off and the pairs move from the larger group in order to sit together. Each pair then discusses what, if any, religious beliefs the pair have. No pressure should be put on the pairs to disclose things that they are not happy to disclose but an atmosphere should have been created prior to doing this activity that encourages participants to share their views.

After about 10 minutes, the pairs reconvene to form the larger group. The facilitator encourages a feedback and discussion session.

Evaluation activity

Each person, in turn, says what he or she found most and least useful about the activity.

Activity 3

Aim of the activity

To explore the concept of 'God'.

Environmental requirements

A circle of chairs in a large room in which participants can pair off for the activity. Alternatively, a series of small rooms can be used for the pairs work and the group can reconvene in the larger.

Number in group

Between 5 and 20 participants

Process

The group divides into small groups of two or three people. Each group 'brainstorms' words or phrases that they associate with the word God. These comments are jotted down onto flipchart sheets. After fifteen minutes, the larger group reconvenes and a plenary session is held in which students discuss their comments.

Evaluation activity

Each person, in turn, says what he or she found most and least useful about the activity.

Activity 4

Aim of the activity

To examine atheism and agnosticism.

Environmental requirements

A circle of chairs in a large room in which participants can pair off for the activity. Alternatively, a series of small rooms can be used for the pairs work and the group can reconvene in the larger.

Number in group

Between 5 and 20 participants

Process

The group divides into pairs. Each pair sits opposite one another and discusses what the words atheism and agnosticism mean to them. They are allowed to make any comments at all, descriptive, analytical or critical. After ten minutes, the larger group reconvenes and a discussion is held about the pairs activity.

Evaluation activity

Each person, in turn, says what he or she found most and least useful about the activity.

Activity 5

Aim of the activity

To explore the relationship between spirituality and nursing.

Environmental requirements

A circle of chairs in a large room in which participants can pair off for the activity. Alternatively, a series of small rooms can be used for the pairs work and the group can reconvene in the larger.

Number in group

Between 5 and 20 participants

Process

The group divides into groups of four or five. Each group discusses how spirituality relates (or does not relate) to a particular aspect of nursing: children's nursing, oncology, care of the elderly, mental health and so forth. Comments from each group are jotted down on flip chart sheets. After fifteen minutes, the larger group reconvenes, the flip charts are talked through and a discussion is held about the relevance or otherwise of spirituality in nursing.

Evaluation activity

Each person, in turn, says what he or she found most and least useful about the activity.

Activity 6

Aim of the activity

To explore 'difficult' questions in nursing practice.

Environmental requirements

A circle of chairs in a large room in which participants can pair off for the activity. Alternatively, a series of small rooms can be used for the pairs work and the group can reconvene in the larger.

Number in group

Between 5 and 20 participants

Process

The group divides into pairs. Each pair nominates one of them as 'A' and the other as 'B'. 'A', then asks the following questions of 'B' as if 'A' were a patient and 'B' were a nurse. 'B' then does his or her best to answer the questions. The participants should be encouraged to take time over this activity and to try out a variety of answers.

- 'Do you believe in God?'
- 'Do you think that believing in God would help me?'
- 'How?'
- 'Would you pray for/with me?'
- 'What do you think will happen to me after I die?'
- 'Why do you think that this has happened to me?'

After about half an hour, the pairs swop roles and 'B' asks the questions of 'A'. Again, each is in the role of 'nurse' and 'patient' and all students should try to respond as naturally and as truthfully as possible.

After a further half an hour, the larger group reconvenes and a discussion is held about how best such questions might be answered. It should be stressed that there are no particular 'right' ways of answering them.

Evaluation activity

Each person, in turn, says what he or she found most and least useful about the activity.

Activity 7

Aim of the activity

To explore values clarification.

Environmental requirements

A circle of chairs in a large room in which participants can pair off for the activity. Alternatively, a series of small rooms can be used for the pairs work and the group can reconvene in the larger.

Number in group

Between 5 and 20 participants

Process

Each student is given a copy of the Spiritual Values Clarification Questionnaire which appears as Appendix III in this book. Each is asked to take about 15 minutes to complete the questionnaire and is reminded that there are no 'right' answers but that each item should be completed. After fifteen minutes (or when each student has completed filling in the questionnaire) the lecturer or facilitator works through each item and encourages a discussion about the various responses.

Evaluation activity

Each person, in turn, says what he or she found most and least useful about the activity.

8 Concluding dialogue

In this final chapter, we review the study through a conversation. A study of this sort cannot offer definite answers and it can only be hoped that it adds to the continuing debate on an important but delicate topic.

PB. Looking back over the study, what are you views on it at this point?

JH. I think there are some issues that I still need to clarify for myself and possibly work with in the clinical areas. I'm still not totally clear as to the difference between psychological needs and spiritual needs and when I lead discussions about spirituality, I find it difficult to differentiate between the two.

PB. Do you think that matters?

JH. Perhaps, not, as long as spiritual issues are raised and debated. However, one half of me thinks that when I am discussing it with students who are confronting spirituality for the first time, to try to differentiate it from the psychological may be helpful. But the other half of me wonders if I am making too much of it. Perhaps it should be something we just discuss and the outcome is going to be different for each individual. Some groups, I find, can discuss spirituality quite openly and can grasp particular spiritual needs quite quickly while others take it very slowly. Some can get quite angry because they don't seem to grasp the relevance of it. But then maybe it is the first time that they have confronted the topic and they may be wanting *answers* and that things aren't black and white in this field. Perhaps they have to go through that doubt and anger before they get to more of an understanding.

PB. I was wondering as you were talking about whether or not its got anything to with the age of the students.

JH. I don't necessarily think so, because some older students have found it quite difficult and have been angry and younger ones have accepted spirituality. You may expect that the younger ones would find it more difficult because they may not have confronted spirituality before or not had as many life experiences.

PB There are a couple of points that I feel about that. I have noticed with my own students - particularly undergraduates, the younger students, that many more of them profess to be Christians nowadays. Whereas, when I first became a nurse teacher, that would not have been the case. I wonder if spirituality and religion go in cycles and that at the moment, we are seeing something of what might be called a 'revivalist' spirit? What are your thoughts about that?

JH. I wouldn't say that there have been a large number of 'born again' Christians in the groups but what I have noticed is that issues about life and things that are happening in the world - for example Somalia, Bosnia - they have been used as points for discussion, for example 'Why is there so much famine in Somalia? and 'Why are the Yugoslavs killing each other?' Perhaps people are looking now for answers for 'why' things are happening.

PB. Haven't they always done that and hasn't religion, traditionally, been the source of answers or at least of comfort? It often struck me during the study, that a number of the respondents related spirituality to some sort of security and I wonder if the sorts of questions you are finding in your students are the age old ones that have more traditionally been addressed to the clergy? In other words, are teachers who facilitate groups about spirituality, stepping into the shoes of the clergy, at least to some degree? Or is that too pretentious an idea? It may even be a dangerous one.

JH. It is difficult for me to judge that because I have only been addressing these issues with students for the past year. So whether they've being doing this before, I can't tell. There haven't been any studies, to my knowledge, that have examined students' perceptions of spirituality. But also, alongside that, maybe we ought to investigate patients and clients spirituality and to what extent they use their spirituality to cope with their condition or illness. There seem to be very few British studies that investigate this. And the question could be asked 'is it right for educationalists to be leading discussions about spirituality when it may not be relevant to patients' conditions?'

PB. But didn't we find that most of the respondents in this study, felt that spirituality *was* relevant to patient care? I suppose that's not really the point, though. The point is, as you say, to find out whether or not *patients* feel the need for spiritual sustenance. I know there have been a variety of American studies about patients' perceptions of the spiritual but I agree that there seem to be few British studies to date. Whether or not there would be significant differences between the two cultures remains an open question. What would be more revealing, perhaps, would be to make cross cultural comparisons between East and West for I know that, for example, the Muslim faith has a very significant part to play in patients' experience of their condition. Exactly how you would carry out a study of that sort, I am not sure.

JH. That, perhaps, leads onto the question about nurses opening up patient's spiritual concerns and then not having the skills to deal with whatever happens. And I have a worry that some nurses following these sessions may feel they are experts at dealing with spiritual issues but deal inappropriately with whatever happens.

PB. Yes. I think that is a really important point. I think it is the sort of dilemma that faces any nurse teacher who runs courses of this sort. That includes courses on counselling, handling aggression and, in fact, any sort of experiential workshop. The danger must always be that short courses merely scratch the surface: they don't get at the deeper skills that are needed. On the other hand, I have a suspicion that all this is not about skills in the end. In the end, I suspect that it is more about sustaining relationships with patients and being able to cope with the total relationship. I have found in other studies that nurses seem to put a high premium on the personal qualities of the nurse rather than on any skills that she or he may have. However, all this does not really get round the problem that you raised: that students may be a bit cavalier in dealing with patient's spiritual problems. On the other hand, do you think that patient's are likely to open up in this way to young students?

JH. In my experience, and from what students have told me, if those students have built up a rapport and relationship with their patients, then they may very well open up and talk about spiritual issues. I may be doing the students a disservice by saying they may tend to dive in without thinking but many students have said that they feel comfortable, on one level, with discussing these issues but if they get in too deep, they wish to call in someone else to help them but are unsure as to who this other person should be. In a general hospital setting, I am not sure who this could be because counsellors and psychologists are not readily available and I am reluctant to say 'chaplain' because they may not always be the most appropriate person.

PB. I would say that neither might counsellors or psychologists be the appropriate people and that raises the question of 'who is?' Perhaps, this is just the point: that we are *all* the appropriate people to talk about these issues. Certainly during this study, from the point of view of the literature and of the comments made by respondents, it has become clear that spiritual issues are fairly fundamental ones and ones that are addressed, at some point, by almost everyone. Perhaps, then, we need not look for 'experts'. On the other hand, one intuitively feels that this could also be a dangerous path. I know from counselling, that people really can get in too deep. I would imagine that this is even more likely in the spiritual domain. After all, who has the ultimate answers in this field? I suppose, though, we have to start somewhere. People *do* want to talk about spiritual issues and I know from experience that the very fact of being able to do so makes a difference. It may not be a question of being particularly skilled or very knowledgeable but more a case of allowing people your *time*.

JH. If spiritual needs are to do with giving love, receiving love, the need for hope and forgiveness, then that is to do with the presence of the nurse and her attitude rather than her counselling skills.

PB. So it has a lot to do with the student's attitude towards talking about spiritual matters?

JH. And their ability to care for their patients. So spirituality becomes an integral part of the nurse's role rather than some 'extra special'.

PB. Are you saying that, in the past, you feel it has been treated as something 'extra special' and not necessarily incorporated into the nurse's everyday role?

JH. Yes. The spiritual needs of a Muslim would, perhaps, be seen that they have special food or time for prayers and meditation and I consider that nurses have seen that as an 'extra' rather than as an expression of that patient's spirituality. It is something 'extra' rather than being an integral part of care.

PB. Whereas, for the patient - especially, perhaps, for the Muslim, the whole issue of spirituality is central. I feel you are right: if nurses really do want to care for the whole person, then they have to look after spiritual needs in a 'deeper' sense than just working through certain rituals that they have learned about 'looking after people from different cultures'. On the other hand, this is quite a tall order. In order to learn about all of the main religions of the worlds, students (and teachers) would have to do a lot of learning. I think this is where travel comes into the picture and why it is gratifying to see and increasing interest in transcultural aspects of care. As nurses travel more widely and more easily, I feel that they may probably get a deeper sense of some of these spiritual issues, although I am not suggesting that this will necessarily happen automatically. You can quite easily travel with your eyes shut.

JH. Don't you think that nurse education should take more of a multicultural perspective about issues and maybe incorporate some philosophy into the curriculum?

PB. By that, do you mean philosophy in the sense of, for example, 'eastern philosophy'? Or do you mean philosophy in a more general, academic sense?

JH. Perhaps both. That may help students feel more comfortable in discussing issues in which there are no definite answers. One of the things we all find difficult is the idea of discussing issues to which there are no definite answers.

PB. That, of course, could be said to be a Western view, in itself. If we were Muslims, for example, we *would* have definite answers. This may also be the case with some of the fundamentalist Christian sects who would also argue, presumably, that there are Biblical answers to most things.

This study has made me think a lot about both spiritual issues and about how we teach in this domain. What do you feel should happen next?

JH. I certainly think that there should be more research in this field, both in terms of nurses and finding out what patients feel. I think there is a lot more work to be done from a nurse education point of view but I feel, as nurses, we should go out into the clinical areas and try dealing with spiritual issues on a day to day basis. There is no point in teaching something unless it is feasible and realistic in clinical practice.

PB. One other point that struck me a number of times during the study, was how often spirituality was linked to religion and to God. I quite like the idea of spirituality being a broader sort of concept and one that involves searching for meaning. Also, as we have gathered from the literature, the concept of religion does not automatically include a concept of God. I was thinking of the work of Paul Tillich, in particular, here. Perhaps we have to broaden out our thinking about the spiritual and then we will be able to make it more pragmatic, as you suggest.

JH. I wholeheartedly agree. It is vital that nurses believe all patients have a spiritual dimension rather than just consider those that are religious.

Appendix I
Example interview schedule

Introduction
- Explanation about the study.
- Explanation about the tape and its relevance.
- Give format of interview.
- Stress confidentiality.
- Stress no right or wrong answers.
- Stress no rush.

Background Details
- Length of time working in clinical
  area.
- Grade.
- Responsibilities.
- Age.
- Year qualified.

Main Issues
- Understanding of Spirituality.
- Influences.

Professional awareness of patients spiritual needs.
- Assessment of spiritual needs.

- Meeting patients spiritual needs.
- Thoughts and feelings relating to the 'why?' of an illness.
- Personal thoughts and feelings relating to meaning and purpose of life
- Sources of hope, love, trust, sense of forgiveness.
- Sources of strength.
- Meaning of God.
- Relevance of religion.
- Thoughts and feelings relating to own mortality.
- Awareness of own spiritual needs.
- Any further points
- Thank respondent

Appendix II
Annotated interview
transcripts

Two annotated transcripts are offered here. They illustrate, partly, the process of analysing interview transcripts in qualitative research but they offer, also, a commentary on the interviews as they unfold. The aim of such transcription is not to interpret the interviews but to begin to summarise some of the issues.

The first interview was conducted with a person who worked in a health care setting where spirituality was an important part of the philosophy of care.

Interview one

Researcher   So can you just tell me how long you've been working here?

Respondent   Yes, about 2½ years.

Researcher   And so what is your contact with the clients or patients that you have here?

Respondent   Well, the first contact most patients have here is with the telephones and they will phone up and more often than not, a friend phones up first of all. Eventually they will phone up - the patient - and we often have very long discussions with them or they could phone up in great distress to start off with so it varies actually, just the amount of contact you have with the patient in the first instance. But usually they make the phone call and we tell them all about the centre and then they take it from there whether they want to come in or not.

Researcher   Right, as you know I'm doing this research interview into spirituality and I just want to find out - what does spiritual or spirituality mean to you?

Respondent   Well, I think it is addressing the inner need that we all have[1] and there comes a point when you recognise it and I suppose that for me happened when I was 36. And up to that point, I hadn't recognised what that inner need[2] was although looking back I suppose I could say my life was always very happy and I would have thought I had everything. But there was always an unfulfilled need and a need that made me feel guilty at times because I couldn't quite put my finger on why I wasn't as happy as I should have been, having a happy marriage and a nice home, two lovely children[3]. So I should have had everything but there was just something missing and I never knew what it was, until I found my own spirituality within me and that fulfilled the need and I suddenly realised[4].

Researcher   So what made you realise that?

---

[1] Spirituality refers to an 'inner need' that appears to be in everyone.

[2] Unrecognised inner need, until the age of 36. Note that Jung (1984) suggested that spiritual concerns tend to be raised in the second half of a person's life.

[3] There was a feeling of unrecognised need, although 'external' situation seemed happy.

[4] Spirituality fulfilled a need. It satisfied something that was 'missing'.

Respondent   Well, I think that that is going to be different for everybody[5] you ask and for many people I think it can come about as a crisis situation[6] in their life especially for people who come here. They find their spirituality through the crisis of having cancer[7]. It could have been any other illness; it could be a bereavement[8].

Researcher   What about for you, if that's not too personal?

Respondent   No, it's not personal[9]. For me, it was something difficult to define in words because it was something over and above something that actually happened to me, in the sense that I'm saying to you, having an illness or a bereavement; it was something more subjective which is rather strange and difficult to understand[10]. It was a feeling (pause) that something was going to happen and that went on for quite a long time and I didn't know what it was and then, I suppose... I think the catalyst was my Grandmother dying perhaps, and I wondering about things and then my sister-in-law giving me a book called "Life After Death"[11]. So I read the book and I realised there was a whole load of questions that this book

---

[5] Recognition of spiritual need can be different for everyone.

[6] For many, it comes through a crisis.

[7] 'Spirituality through having cancer'.

[8] Not necessarily cancer: it could be any other illness or bereavement.

[9] Corrects researcher: not too personal. Reminiscent of Roger's point (1964) that 'what is most personal is most general'. The personal issues are also the universal ones.

[10] Strange and difficult to define. Struggles to find words to express feelings and thoughts.

[11] Book helped respondent to make sense of what was happening.

didn't ask and it set me off on search[12]. At that point, I didn't even know I was looking for spirituality but I did start looking... for answers to our reason to be and what life was all about[13]. It only came about some months later when I really got into looking, that it evolved, it happened, and I think this is very, very natural and very, very necessary for when you start opening up - what I would call becoming seeking, seeking the truth[14]. I think there are a lot of people who seek the truth but they don't actually open up the spiritual aspect of themselves and when they don't, that is when they can get into a lot of trouble because it should actually - it's like a flower opening - happens very naturally[15]. It did for me and I had no idea because I hadn't even looked into it. I didn't have any understanding at that time but it did happen naturally and to me, it is something that can never be forced[16]. However much I go on about talking to anyone about what happens to me, it can never happen to them because it happened to me[17]. It happens to them because it is right for them not because I'm telling them about me[18].

Researcher   We'll perhaps come back to you personally a little bit more

---

[12] Began a search.

[13] Began search for answer to question: 'What is life all about?'.

[14] Involved seeking for the truth.

[15] The respondent feels that a lot of people ignore the spiritual side of themselves. Can cause a lot of trouble but it is a 'natural' process. If it *is* a 'natural process', is the assumption that it will happen to *everyone*? This has not been the argument so far.

[16] Something that cannot be forced.

[17] A personal and idiosyncratic process.

[18] It has to be right for the individual. You cannot generalise from your own experience. In a sense, though, this is what the respondent may be doing.

in a minute but I just want to relate this now to where you work[19]. How important do you think this notion of spirituality is to your work here at the centre?

Respondent   It's very, very important and I think you will find that it is quite a unique place in as much as the majority of the people who work here, will have found this also. We are all on the same wavelength - there aren't many people who haven't, and it is the heart of the centre[20]. And why I think it is important, because as I talk to a lot of patients particularly when they do start asking about this sort of aspect of the work here. When they do, we can have a talk about it because in my belief and my understanding and in what I have come to learn here, it is the heart of the matter and it's the heart of the healing programme that we do here. We offer people what I call keys to different doors[21]. But it's up to them whether they go through them or not. It's their choice, there is no pressure but they are on offer and it is this crucial door of one's spirituality that to me is the essence of how well they are going to become and can get. This is the point where if they decide to go down this avenue they have got everything possible and open to them. Without it, I think it's rare that somebody could really make a good recovery because we are leaving out the essential part of ourselves[22], that aspect of ourselves. Most healing goes on, as far as I can understand, at that deep level. It filters through all the different levels of our being[23] until it gets to the physical. There is no reason for the physical to

---

[19] Researcher moves away from the 'personal' to the world of work.

[20] Like-minded colleagues. Alludes to 'everyone feeling the same way'. Not necessarily clear *what* everyone feels.

[21] A healing programme and the 'key to doors'. It is not clear to what this metaphor of 'doors' refers.

[22] Spirituality seems to be a key to recovery.

[23] Levels of being referred to but not made explicit.

138

be out of balance[24] if you have every other part of you in balance. Leaving it out, you are maybe curing something temporary but will come back again because you haven't got the heart of the matter[25].

Researcher   So you're giving them the key here, to the spiritual.

Respondent   Yes, I mean people don't come here long enough for anything other, they do it themselves[26]. People will be here to teach them either for the one day or for the week. If they come for a week, then they have a little longer. But it is a pathway, it opens up doors and it is up to them whether they want to pursue it[27]. What they do and how they do it is purely up to them and everybody will do it differently, but if they do go down that path, they really are going on a journey of self discovery[28].

Researcher   So have you been aware, while you've been working at the centre, that people/patients/clients that they've got this spiritual need?

Respondent   I think that we've all got it[29] but we don't all recognise it or

---

[24] The issue of 'physical balance' is raised. Further, the idea that the 'physical' will not be out of balance if 'every other part is in balance'. The respondent does not elaborate on the question of what counts as 'the other part'.

[25] Again, spirituality seems to be at 'the heart of the matter'.

[26] Seems to be suggesting that *all* patients seek the spiritual.

[27] Metaphors of pathways and doors. Also, respondent suggests that final decisions are always up to the patients.

[28] Process involves self-discovery.

[29] Reiterates universality of the idea of spiritual need.

we don't need to recognise it[30]. As I said before, it usually takes something that hit us between the eyes before we wake up because if your life is wonderful and happy why bother? Unless like in my case, it became something that went on in my mind more or less[31].

Researcher   So what kind of spiritual needs did those people have that you've met. Can you describe them?

Respondent   That's a difficult one to put into words[32]. I suppose our needs are all the same, there isn't anybody that has a different need than another in the spiritual sense and wanting to become whole, wanting to make that connection with ourselves, that deeper inner connection[33]. It's there and even when we don't recognise it, we are trying to fulfil that need perhaps in more of an earthy way we become obsessed about something we put all our heart and passion in anything like maybe playing golf to perfection which is an impossibility obviously. It could be anything that you do to an extent because that gives you a real purpose and aim[34], that when you think about it, it can't go on forever can it? You can't be forever wanting to knock a little ball into a little hole -what is

---

[30] Reiterates non-recognition by some people of their inherent need for the spiritual.

[31] Two possibilities seem to present themselves: the crisis situation, which leads to recognition of spiritual needs or a more cognitive approach to identifying the need.

[32] Difficulty of finding words to describe spiritual needs.

[33] All spiritual needs are the same: all involve the person in seeking wholeness.

[34] Gives purpose and aim to the person.

the point in that?[35]

Researcher   Do you assess on an individual level, do you assess people's individual spiritual needs?

Respondent   No, it's very much unsaid. We do have healing on offer here and it is purely their choice whether they want to take that up or not[36]. Very few people refuse it, most people enjoy the experience enormously and then go on to find a healer where they live to carry that on but very often it's a first experience for them and I think that is the time when they discover certain peace - not always but it's different for everyone[37].

Researcher   So am I right in saying that you attempt to help people meet their spiritual needs perhaps through healing?

Respondent   Yes, it is through healing.

Researcher   And is that the only way?

Respondent   Basically here it is a key. Again it's something that can't be spoken of in the same way as you could speak of "let's get our emotions under control"[38]. It's not quite like that because

---

[35] Seems to suggest that 'ordinary' activities are not enough. There must be something 'more'. There is a sense, here, that day-to-day activities may lead to a sense of futility and a need for something more.

[36] Patients have choice about whether or not to accept healing.

[37] Few refuse healing, most enjoy it and seek out a 'local' healer. Question: are the patients in a position to refuse?

[38] Difficult, again, to put into words. Ineffable. A *mystical* experience, perhaps. William James (1902) suggested that mystical experiences had at least four qualities: ineffability (an indescribable quality); noetic quality (mysterious knowing, or knowing beyond the inputs from the senses); transiency and passivity on the part of the person having the experience. In some senses, James' qualities are tautological.

it has to come from within the need of the actual recognising that you want to look for something over and above, what ever else is going on in your life. As I said, it is something that blossoms, maybe that you will read a book and you'll think, yes, I can understand that book, but as I did, there are lots of questions now and I want answers[39]. So the more you read, the more questions and you can't stop in the end, you have to go on[40]. But you can always get answers and for me, I don't think there is a question you can ask for which there is no answer[41]. The question is, does one understand the answers?[42]

Researcher   When you try and fathom the way of an illness or suffering, because you see a lot here, what thoughts and feelings are conjured up for you?

Respondent   Well, I don't actually have to do that because I don't work in that aspect with the patients so it isn't something that I sit and ponder over in any professional sense. But I can only answer for myself, how I feel personally that I think probably we all recreate for ourselves our own reality so everything we have experienced, we have actually created. Through the creation of what we've done, maybe we can learn from that and it can

---

[39] Desire for answers.

[40] Impelled to go on in the search for answers.

[41] Suggests that there are no questions that do not have answers. Link this to the work of the logical positivists who would argue that it does not follow that because we can *phrase* a question that there is necessarily an answer. It is easy to phrase questions to which there are no answers. Absurd examples, to make the point, might include: 'why are swans green?' or 'what is the meaning of iron?'

[42] It is a question of *understanding* the answers.

be very painful[43]. So it's not something that you actually can say "here comes somebody, I think they've got this illness because of" - you don't know that, you don't know why[44]. You have to be very careful because you also can actually make somebody feel that it is their fault, so this is a very dangerous area really but I think again, only when you've really looked into this and come to really good understanding to what life is all about, can you actually look at that and say "well, I can see why I may have created this or I may have taken it on"[45]. Because my own belief is that we have many, many lives, different bodies[46], but the essence is within us, we come again and again until we become so perfected, we don't need to come again and this particular life, any particular life, yes we have this and this and this is going to happen and maybe we've actually taken on that before in order that we learn these particular lessons or it could be that because of whatever we do, every cause has an effect so whatever we do, we are creating an effect somewhere[47]. It may not manifest in this life, but probably in the future world[48]. And so, very often the cause of an illness, in my understanding, would be deep down. It could be simply that you have had the most horrendous experience and unable to deal with that experience at an emotional level and blocked it

---

[43] Life experiences can be painful.

[44] May ponder on 'reason' for patient's illness.

[45] Important not to 'blame' people for their illness. On the other hand, respondent seems to be alluding to possible causes within the self.

[46] Belief system included notion of 'many lives and many bodies'.

[47] Beliefs seem to link to Buddhist ideas and to Chaos theory. See, for example (Ferguson 1976; Ferruci 1982; Goleman 1972; Tart 1975).

[48] Notion of 'future world' raised here.

	off and there it is, deep down inside you[49]. That could manifest. It's always there until it's dealt with whatever life time and eventually in one life, "look I'm going to deal with this", and it will eventually filter through into the physical because I see it as a blockage, an energy blockage.
Researcher	Perhaps you've answered this question but I'll put it again. When you question the meaning of life or the purpose of life for yourself, what beliefs or convictions strike you most clearly or deeply?
Respondent	Again, I would say it evolved over some years now - about nine years. So the whole thing has evolved and you don't read one or two books and think yes, this is my truth". It isn't your truth, it's the person who has written the book - it's their truth. And I have no way of knowing and I couldn't say I believed in it. Conviction comes from within yourself and that took a few years to get the conviction through all sorts of experiences and what happened to me and what happened to me[50] on my pathway. Eventually, I came to my own conviction within myself so that I could say "this is my belief, my understanding". I wouldn't say I wouldn't ever change that because it's possible but I can't see how[51]. I think I could improve upon it but when I say I believe that life goes on, that's from my own experiences, from my own understanding and I wouldn't expect anyone to believe it because I think they'd be fools to believe it because I said so.

---

[49] Illness may be linked to problems 'deep down' in the person's life or being.

[50] Truth does not lie in books but comes from personal experience and personal conviction.

[51] Likely that belief system will not change further.

Go out and have your own experiences, find out the truth for yourself because if you start asking questions, you get the answers[52].

Researcher   So what is your source of strength? Is it this belief in truth?

Respondent   Yes, my belief in the universal power of love[53]. Some people would call that God, some people would call it divinity. Whatever, there are all sorts of names for it, it doesn't really matter. To me, it's not a personality, it's not a little old man sitting in a rocking chair or anything like that[54]. It is this all knowing power. And I have that understanding and it makes everybody here seem rather very small in comparison to it. You know, it's something that is very humbling to recognise and to know that life has a purpose[55], that's very important. I used to think, well I used to get out of a lot of things by saying "who cares - so what if I fail, it doesn't matter, I shall be dead one day, so what, that's the end of everything". And I used to get out of a lot of things that way, but you can't get out of anything once you change your ideas. So for me, it is a reason to be. It gives me my purpose in life, a reason to be[56], to know that whatever one suffers here is all for a good cause in the end and to keep on keeping on.

Researcher   You mentioned God and the next question I was going to ask you is how far do religious affiliations seem to be a source of strength for you?

---

[52] Seems to suggest that if you ask the right questions, the answers will 'emerge'. How this happens is not made explicit.

[53] Universal power of love. Not described in further detail.

[54] God is not 'the old man in the sky'. Instead, God is 'this all knowing power'.

[55] Life has a purpose.

[56] The spiritual gives a meaning to life, a 'reason to be'.

Respondent	Well, I was born and brought up in the Church of England and didn't mean a lot to me actually[57]. I was even confirmed and I thought "what a waste of time". It meant nothing to me but now I can take out the good and put aside the dogma and that' fine. I can enjoy going to a church service - I really enjoy it now. I feel I can go into any church and into any temple[58] and I could actually go into and get exactly the same because a church is a church and a temple is a temple. Basically you don't need to go anywhere because you can find that temple within yourself[59]. But as for religions, they are all stepping stones along the way as far as I can see and each one has been infiltrated by mans' ideas and hence the dogma. So they are all stepping stones along the way but they all lead to the top of the mountain[60].
Researcher	And so I was going to say could you explain in a few sentences what God means to you, but is God like the top of the mountain?[61]
Respondent	Absolutely, not that we would ever get to there - He is way above the top of the mountain or He/She/It. The power is just all pervading[62]. It would get too complicated to explain it really but I think from what I have understood, where we stand in the world is not the be all and end all. There are many other spheres way over and above us which we can

---

[57] Organised Church meant little to the respondent.

[58] Can go into any 'church or temple'.

[59] No need to go anywhere: the temple is within.

[60] Further metaphors: stepping stones leading to the top of the mountain. The metaphor occurs frequently in the literature on *psychosynthesis*. See, for example, Ferruci 1982 and Tart 1975.

[61] Researcher appears to try to make the metaphor more concrete.

[62] All pervading power *above* the mountain, world, universe.

actually one day go to[63]. For my understanding, we actually set out from a point as a tiny spark and eventually found our way, and we say down because we speak in linear time, and as we came down, we were clothed in whatever, in the substance of where we were at. Until eventually, we come into the earth and were clothed with this physical body but it actually covers various bodies on the way down from where we started out. And the idea is to go there and back again, it is a conscious being and we then discard these layers as we go back up. Where we actually go back up to is not the highest.

Researcher   So where is the highest?

Respondent   Well from my understanding, you can go a lot higher into other realms[64] which we are not capable of going into simply because we are where we came from, you cannot go beyond

---

[63] There are other spheres that we can go to, above the current one.

[64] Many of the ideas that this respondent discusses have things in common with *theosophy*. In a discussion of the principles of theosophy (an organisation founded in New York, in 1875, by the Russian clairvoyant, Helena Petrovna Blavatsky), Hinnels (1984) describes the some of the principles of theosophy thus:

(for the theosophist) the universe consists of seven interpenetrating 'planes'; each of us, accordingly, has seven bodies (Divine, Spiritual, Intuitional, Etheric, Physical), the first three comprising the 'Ego' or 'Overself', which reincarnates countless times, experiencing *karma* (happiness and suffering as results of good and evil actions) and evolving towards full 'Selfhood' in conscious cooperation with the divine purpose...Members are encouraged to practice meditation but no particular religious practice is enjoined (Hinnels 1984: 328).

It would, of course, be wrong to assume that the respondent was necessarily describing a theosophical point of view but it is interesting to note some of the similarities in thinking.

where we came from[65]. But it gets rather complicated to go further onto there but I don't actually hold with the fact that we are divine beings because we are not. I just feel that we are spiritual beings[66].

Researcher   Now if you had spent some time considering your own mortality, and perhaps you've answered this, what strong thoughts and feelings about it do you have? You don't have to answer it if you haven't perhaps considered your own mortality or if it's too painful?

Respondent   Well, my own mortality is something that I really look forward to the day I die - one half of me[67]. I really think that's going to be a wonderful adventure. One half of me can't wait to go, I find living here very difficult in a lot of ways and I really long, long, long to go to the point where - when that energy is out of balance, I suppose it goes back to that time when I said I wasn't fulfilled and what was that feeling but you have to get that energy into balance and use it[68]. Basically I've learnt that it has to be used, so it's sort of just leaving it sort of around this area, churning area of the body to use it so that life is more fulfilling and you get the most out of life. So the other half of me says "gosh, I'd hate to go anywhere because I really enjoy life" but there's this other half that says that there's this other place better than this and this is where it's difficult.

Researcher   So you're certainly not frightened of it?

---

[65] Complicated: we cannot go beyond where we came from.

[66] People are spiritual beings.

[67] Looks forward to own mortality. Another side of the person.

[68] Need to get energy balance right. The respondent is not specific about the nature of this *energy* as used in this context.

Respondent	No not at all[69]. Not in a sense as I'm sitting here. I'm not going to die tomorrow or as far as I know. I mean, one may start to have that, you really can't be sure how one would feel confronted with it but there is a part of me that looks forward to that.
Researcher	So how do you meet your spiritual needs? If you could sum that up? If you do meet them, do you meet them to any degree?
Respondent	Working towards - no, I don't feel I meet them totally. Only when I feel, there are sometimes when one finds that total inner peace, but that's not always possible to feel that all the time[70].
Researcher	When do you feel that?
Respondent	Working really[71].
Researcher	Do you mean here?
Respondent	Yes, working sort of on that level - in that way. That's one way of meeting those needs. I don't think it's a case of going down on your knees and that sort of thing. That doesn't, although sitting quietly it goes a long way to meeting those needs obviously[72]. But it's like everything. Having everything in balance, a time for work, a time for prayer, a time for finding the peace basically. It's taken me a long time

---

[69] Not frightened of death.

[70] Need to find inner peace as a means of satisfying spiritual needs and the problem of not being able to meet them all the time.

[71] Peace can come through work.

[72] Sitting quietly can help satisfy spiritual needs. T.S. Eliot: 'Teach us to care and not to care. Teach us to sit still.'

to get to this point and all that time, you've got a lot of unanswered questions you can't find that inner peace but you're working towards it. It's an ongoing thing - you can't leave it alone and you can't go backwards. This is it, it does change your life once you start on this pathway of searching and seeking and so on, you can't go back. You can't jump off the escalator or go back down it because it will keep on carrying you up.[73]

Researcher   So it is like a quest?

Respondent   Yes, it is[74].

Researcher   And so there's nothing specifically, or no four or five things that actually helped you me those needs? What you're saying, it's a balance between...

Respondent   It is a balance[75]. I suppose being with other people, who are like minded is very necessary. Sitting quietly, either in a sort of contemplation prayer, meditation whatever you like is very important and putting it into your daily work, putting it into your life. In fact the whole point of it is I suppose is simply being what you believe. It's o.k. to read as many books as you like but if you don't put that into action, you may as well throw those books out of the window. They're not doing you any good. So in actual fact, is to live your belief[76]. Does that make any sense?

Researcher   Yes, I think so.

---

[73] Metaphor of travelling up an escalator. You can't go back down, you can only go further up.

[74] The process is like a quest.

[75] Reaffirms need for balance. But a balance between *what* and *what*?

[76] Need to live your belief.

150

Respondent	So that you don't actually need to say it to anybody. You don't need to speak to somebody in the general sense because you are that. You don't have to say something to say to somebody "well, these are my beliefs and this is the way I think I should be" because it just comes across[77].
Researcher	And I suppose the fact that you know it within you, does that help?
Respondent	Well, that's where you find the core of inner peace: its that you know that you're not struggling on your own. That you know that, well you've got to put out the thought of please help me and that help is there - that because this isn't all there is, that you have got help if you recognise it, it makes life such easier. To feel, "well, I'm really not quite so alone as I thought I was, I really don't have to struggle". I don't know how many people can really get through the traumas of life if they are really an island just to themselves. I really don't know how they do it. I feel for them because I couldn't, I really couldn't. As I said, when life is swinging along, it's wonderful, you don't have to worry. It's when it gets difficult, people think "well, why me?". So five things are probably too many.
Researcher	I don't think there's anything else I specifically want to ask you. Is there anything else you want to add to what I've said or what you've said or anything else?
Respondent	Well. I just think there's many ways up the mountain and it's up to each one to choose and find a way that suits them. People working here come from all different types of religious backgrounds and we have all different types of religion working here and it's lovely because we're all in harmony, it's really nice, but we don't talk about it very much. It's very

---

[77] It should be *evident* that you have spiritual beliefs: you should not, necessarily have to talk about them. Instead, you should be *demonstrating* them.

151

much unspoken but I think a lot of people will walked into this place and sense a lovely atmosphere of some sort of pervading peace and tranquillity. I don't know what it is but maybe that all personifies what we're all trying to do.

Researcher   Perhaps what spirituality is?

Respondent   Maybe that's what it is - sums it up finding your inner peace[78].

---

[78] Spirituality is about finding your own inner peace.

Interview two

This interview was conducted with a trained nurse working in a hospital setting.

Researcher	The first question I'd like to ask you as the research is about spirituality, could you just tell me what you understand by the term 'spiritual' or 'spirituality'?
Respondent	How I see it, it is not relating to one thing it's not a God, it is whatever that person actually believes in[1]. It maybe an afterlife, it may be an object, could be anything that that person has faith in[2]. That's how I see it.
Researcher	How did you actually come by those beliefs?
Respondent	To be honest, I'd always thought of that but I just actually checked it yesterday in the dictionary, about what spirituality was and it didn't actually say, when I actually looked it up it said all about the afterlife which is maybe not what I thought. I thought it was more just somebody's belief in their idol, their God, an object, just what they believed in[3].
Researcher	How did you come by those beliefs before you liked it up in the dictionary?
Respondent	I just think it's what has always been with me really[4]. I mean as far as Church went, I went to Church when I was younger

---

[1] Spirituality doesn't necessarily involve God. Relates more to peoples' own beliefs.

[2] Examples: afterlife or 'whatever they believe in'.

[3] More than 'an idol' or a God. Reiterates that it is 'what people believe in'. No further elaboration.

[4] Respondent had always had certain beliefs.

and I was a Sunday School teacher for a long time, but that wouldn't have swayed me, I think everybody has got something they believe in, but I don't know if it would necessarily be the Church that I believe in[5].

Researcher   So it is something which you have grown up with?

Respondent   Yes.

Researcher   How important do you think is the notion of spirituality to you as a nurse?

Respondent   I think it's important to recognise other people's beliefs, not necessarily my own feelings, but just other people's feelings when I am nursing them which I don't think it's of prime importance in nursing today, I think we look over other things, we forget that[6].

Researcher   So you're saying that you do think it's important?

Respondent   Yes.

Researcher   I want to expand on that a bit more. Why do you think it's important?

Respondent   Because we are trying to educate people to what they would normally do in everyday life and we tend to regard them as patients when they come in. They are in hospital and they must conform to what we want and that's not the idea of hospitalisation, it should be to bring people back to their norm

---

[5] Used to go to Church and was a Sunday School teacher but that 'did not sway' respondent.

[6] It is important to accept individuals' own belief systems. The spiritual domain is sometimes forgotten in nursing today.

not our norm[7]. I think we take a lot of things away from people when they come in and some people's religion - we had a gentleman, his religion was that he didn't mix with other people, he didn't eat with them and he didn't mix with them, and therefore we have to comply with what their wishes are[8].

Researcher My next question was, have you actually been aware of people having, or patients having spiritual needs?

Respondent It is only the ones that are not deviants from the normal which are different - is not your normal C of E[9] or whatever, it's the Asian minorities or - I can't think what this man's religion was but it wasn't normals C of E but they did have special things that they wanted us to do for them.

Researcher So, if you had to describe patient's spiritual needs, how could you describe them?

Respondent I think I would ask them to describe them to be honest[10]. Because I don't think I could describe them because everybody thinks different things and what their spiritual needs would be so I would ask them to describe what they wanted.

Researcher So your saying it's an individual thing?

Respondent Yes, an individual thing[11].

---

[7] It is important that people have their own norms and do not feel compelled to automatically follow others' beliefs.

[8] Description of a patient's behaviour as 'his religion'.

[9] Church of England cited as 'the normal'.

[10] Respondent would ask patient to describe his or her own spiritual needs.

[11] Spiritual needs are 'an individual thing'.

Researcher	So, how would you feel about initiating a conversation with a patient about spiritual needs? Would you be comfortable going up to them and saying "Can you tell me about your spiritual needs?"
Respondent	I do if I do an assessment[12]. I probably take it more into consideration if I know they're going to be of a different religion that I'm used to[13]. I probably would take it more into consideration then. But I normally ask them if they wanted to see the Priest or anything[14]. But if it is an obvious different religion then I would probably go into it a bit more.
Researcher	So you wouldn't feel too uncomfortable about that?
Respondent	No[15].
Researcher	How do you feel about responding to patients if they start initiating a conversation about spirituality?
Respondent	I don't personally mind. I think some people are threatened when people start expressing their spirituality on other people[16] and it's personal - if you do not agree with them it should not be forced upon them, which does sometimes happen with people who have strong religious beliefs[17].
Researcher	If you have identified that anyone's got spiritual needs, do you

---

[12] Spiritual needs are part of initial assessment of patient.

[13] Respondent notes 'different religions'.

[14] Asks if patient would like to see 'the priest'.

[15] Does not feel uncomfortable about talking about spiritual issues with patients.

[16] Some people are threatened by spiritual issues.

[17] People should not force their beliefs on others.

discuss them with anyone on the ward?

Respondent   If there was something they wanted done differently either eating or socialising or doing something on Thursday afternoon different, then we would write it in the assessment then we would talk about it and work toward what they wanted[18].

Researcher   So you would bring it up in report time?

Respondent   Yes.

Researcher   When you personally try and fathom out the why of an illness and suffering, what thoughts and feelings are actually conjured up within you, because you must see quite a bit of suffering in your job[19].

Respondent   I find it quite hard to come to terms with it sometimes, if there is a God why is he letting people go through this?[20] But people's beliefs always stand firm, there was somebody recently who was a gentleman concerned with spirituality and he had every faith as to what was going to happen whereas I couldn't have every faith. He did and no matter what we did his faith was carrying him through to the end[21]. But I find it more difficult to accept what happens to them than they do sometimes.

Researcher   Could you find that a help to you because he could understand, or he had faith?

---

[18] Respondent often relates spiritual issues to *customs* and changes in routine or procedure.

[19] Researcher leads respondent into a discussion of the 'why' of illness.

[20] Why does God allow this to happen?

[21] Example of 'faith being carried through to the end'.

Respondent	I find it quite sad and quite happy[22]. I was happy for him because he had accepted what his fate was going to be, but I was sad for him, I don't know why I was sad for him to accept something which he obviously believed in, but I found it quite sad[23].
Researcher	So it didn't help you really that he had come to terms with his illness?
Respondent	No, it should have done but no it didn't really[24].
Researcher	When you question the meaning of life and the purpose of life for yourself, what beliefs strike you most clearly?
Respondent	I don't know, I always think that we're aiming, something after this life that we're aiming for in this life[25]. At least that's what my Dad always said about the 'goodies', that you have planes of life[26], that you acquire things in this life to go on to the next one. I think it is a trial for what is to come I think[27].
Researcher	What actually gives you hope and trust and a sense of love

---

[22] Situation both 'sad and happy'.

[23] Patient's faith was 'sad'.

[24] Spiritual beliefs did not help patient to come to terms with his illness.

[25] Suggestion of an afterlife.

[26] Reference to father's belief in 'planes of life'. The notions of planes and levels occurs, frequently, in the literature on *transpersonal psychology*. Sometimes described as the 'fourth force' in psychology (after psychodynamic, behavioural and humanistic), transpersonal psychology is concerned with metaphysical beliefs and with 'higher' levels of consciousness. See, for example Tart 1969, 1975; Wallis 1984). The idea also occurs in *theosophy* and other 'mystical' religions (Ferguson 1976).

[27] Life as a trial for what is to come.

and forgiveness in your life?

Respondent   I don't know, I think it's not anything I believe in it's what I see when I'm, nursing, you realise that it's all too short[28] and it doesn't stop the arguing but it stops me walking out on an argument from my house or anything. I would always go back.

Researcher   Why would you go back?

Respondent   Because I couldn't walk out on an argument, I couldn't do that knowing that anything could happen in the hours that we didn't see each other and then I would have to go back and sort it out and be happy with the situation.

Researcher   And does that give you a source of strength do you think? Does your husband - is it your husband your talking about?

Respondent   Yes, or my Mum and Dad.

Researcher   Do they give you a source of strength and hope?

Respondent   Oh yes. I'm, not sure if it's anything spiritual I believe in though[29].

Researcher   You mentioned the planes of life earlier on, does that give you a bit of hope and a bit of strength do you think?

Respondent   It does in the fact that there might be something to follow which we're aiming for, yes. I don't honestly think about it that often[30] because it would probably confuse me as to what I was trying to aim for in this life and whether you actually achieve it or not. But it's reassuring in a way I think you may

---

[28] Life it too short.

[29] Support comes from family and not necessarily from spiritual beliefs.

[30] Respondent doesn't often think about spiritual matters.

need something to believe in because it's the fear of the unknown, of what you might be going into[31].

Researcher I'm trying to identify what your source of strength is in your life. Could you highlight source of strength?

Respondent I don't know. Can you rephrase it?

Researcher Or, when things perhaps aren't going too well for you in whatever, it doesn't have to be illness or suffering but if things aren't going too well, what is it that you might latch onto?

Respondent I just think it will always get better, basically, whatever happens and I think time is my strength because I know that given time it will sort itself out. That's probably my strength[32].

Researcher The next question I was going to ask - how far do religious affiliations in your life seem to be a resource and strength?

Respondent My Dad's quite interested in certain different people's religion and he interests me in the way that they think he's very concerned about Saudi and the Arabs and their sole belief in this one person who will save them all. and he's very interested but he interests me that some people could believe so much, I really wish I could believe so much in one thing but they never falter in that at all. I think it's my Dad, my Dad is interested in a variety of things and he spreads it on to me[33].

Researcher You said you were a Sunday School teacher, how far does that play a part?

---

[31] Belief in 'levels' can be reassuring when faced with the unknown.

[32] Respondent appears to believe in the idea that things will always get better.

[33] Influenced by father's interest in different religions.

160

Respondent	I think it actually made it worse to be honest[34]. It was a quite old fashioned church with everybody over the age of 80 so every week they used to think I was a new member of the Church and I had been going for six years. I'd be greeted as a new member every single week, and I didn't feel after six years that I really belonged somewhere who wouldn't accept me either I was a Sunday School teacher and everything it just sort of drifted away when I did my nurse training[35].
Researcher	So would you say that religious affiliations probably aren't too much of a resource and a strength to you at the moment?
Respondent	Not really, I mean I believe that there is a God[36] but I don't believe that you have to go to Church to be with him or near him, I think you can do it wherever you are, it doesn't really matter where you are. I don't believe you have to go to this big place[37].
Researcher	So in a few sentences could you explain what God is to you?
Respondent	God is just a person the overall, the Maker, he is the overall who gives you choices I think in what life will hold for you and you have to make a choice and you either take the wrong choice or the right choice. It would never be entirely wrong, it may not be the best one but the choices are there which he gives you to choose[38].
Researcher	I think you have answered this, but it you have spent some time considering your own mortality, what strong thoughts or

---

[34] Being a Sunday School teacher 'made things worse'.

[35] Didn't feel accepted as part of the Church.

[36] Believes there is a God.

[37] There is no need to go to church in order to believe in God.

[38] Definition of God, prompted by researcher.

feelings do you have about it?

Respondent   I'd like to think there is another place[39]. To go back a bit,
              you were saying about religious things in maybe the family,
              my Mum had an experience when she was giving birth to me
              or by brother, I can't remember which one, and she saw the
              light[40] and the and she knows someone who has gone
              through that and you realise that there might be something. I
              don't know what it is but there might be something there, and
              that' reassuring to know that somebody's going to be there
              waiting for me[41].

Researcher   So, could that be a source of strength for you?

Respondent   Yes, I think it is[42]. I've never thought about it actually too
              much, at least you know it's not quite the end. I think there is
              something after but now I'm sure there is something after.

Researcher   Are you aware of having any spiritual needs yourself?

Respondent   No. Not really, not that would involve anybody else I don't
              think. Do you know what I mean?[43]

Researcher   It doesn't have to involve anyone else, are there any times or
              any feeling that you perhaps could describe as being spiritual?
              for you?

---

[39] There is 'another place' after death.

[40] Metaphor of 'seeing the light'.

[41] Quotes mother's beliefs but not clear whether or not these are also
respondent's.

[42] Those beliefs are, though, a source of strength.

[43] Not aware of having spiritual needs.

Respondent	I don't really think so, no.
Researcher	Because my next question was are they met to any degree? So you would say that you haven't got a spiritual part to yourself.
Respondent	No, not anything that I would stick to I'm open minded[44].
Researcher	Do you find anything particularly moving, or anything you have to do at some part of the day or some part of the week?
Respondent	No, I find lots of things moving.[45]
Researcher	Can you give me an example?
Respondent	I find groups of people who are doing things together, pulling together, I find that quite emotional whatever it is to do with, it's so emotional that a lot of people could do that altogether and work together, I find that ..
Researcher	So would you mean like a team of people?
Respondent	Yes, or just people who have never met before and they all suddenly join together for one root cause I think that is quite emotional.
Researcher	Can you give me an example of that?
Respondent	Well, I had a cry the other day. A television programme about saving some whales and everybody came out, hundreds and hundreds of people came out to save these whales and they were holding them up in the water for 24 hours., I found that really emotional, all these people holding these whales up. I think what I'm probably getting confused with, you don't

---

[44] No particular 'spiritual part'.

[45] Researcher's intention not clear: appears to have taken up the idea of what might be 'moving' as opposed to staying with the 'spiritual'.

often use the term spirituality, if somebody said that to me straight away I would say religion but it's not religion, it's a much broader thing than religion but when you think of it at first you think of it as a religion but it's not[46].

Researcher   So having perhaps re-defined what you understand by spirituality, because I think initially you said it was perhaps to do with religion, can you redefine it, what it means for you now, now that we have discussed it a bit?[47]

Respondent   I still think it was concerned with some religion, about your attitudes about how your going, I think it's from where you come from and how it all started and events that happened how you foresee why they happened and how you can get over them, and if there is anything in the afterlife it's the whole spirituality, it must be the whole of it as I see it, from the beginning to the end of your life. Whatever you believe in would be included[48].

Researcher   So, just asking you again do you still say now - have you got any spiritual needs yourself do you think?

Respondent   Not a need, I know that there is probably something after but I wouldn't class that as a need, it's just a belief[49].

Researcher   Thank you very much indeed.

---

[46] Emotional experiences can be much broader than religious experiences.

[47] Research is leading a little here and trying to get respondent to redefine responses.

[48] Respondent summarises position on spiritual matters.

[49] Beliefs are more important than spiritual needs.

Appendix III
A spiritual values questionnaire

This questionnaire can be used in a variety of ways. First, in can be used in workshops on spirituality in nursing, with student nurses, to promote discussion. Second, it can be used as a form of *values clarification* to help students to sort out their views on the issue of spirituality and nursing care. Third, it can be used to collect data as part of a research project that explores, further, the concept of spirituality in clinical practice. It should be noted that it is not an *attitudinal* questionnaire. With such instruments, it is usually possible to arrive at an overall score for each respondent (Sommer and Sommer 1991). If this questionnaire is used for research purposes, it is probably best to present only frequency counts of the responses to given items. Whether or not it is used for research purposes, it should be made clear to students that there are no 'right' answers to the items and that they should offer a response to each item.

Students are asked to read each item and to place a tick in the box that follows the item that most closely matches their own view about the item. They should only tick one box for each item.

1. Spirituality is an important aspect of clinical nursing care.

Strongly Agree	Agree	Don't Know	Disagree	Strongly Disagree

2. Generally speaking, patients spiritual needs are met by nursing staff.

Strongly Agree	Agree	Don't Know	Disagree	Strongly Disagree

3. I am clear about my own spiritual values.

Strongly Agree	Agree	Don't Know	Disagree	Strongly Disagree

4. I am clear about my own spiritual needs.

Strongly Agree	Agree	Don't Know	Disagree	Strongly Disagree

5. 'Spirituality' is much the same as 'religion'.

Strongly Agree	Agree	Don't Know	Disagree	Strongly Disagree

6. If you have strong religious beliefs, you should be prepared to share them with others.

Strongly Agree	Agree	Don't Know	Disagree	Strongly Disagree

7. Most religions have a degree of 'truth' in them.

Strongly Agree	Agree	Don't Know	Disagree	Strongly Disagree

8. I would be comfortable talking about spiritual matters with patients.

Strongly Agree	Agree	Don't Know	Disagree	Strongly Disagree

9. Spirituality is a topic that is well covered in our training.

Strongly Agree	Agree	Don't Know	Disagree	Strongly Disagree

10. Most people believe in a God.

Strongly Agree	Agree	Don't Know	Disagree	Strongly Disagree

11. Spirituality is a central part of the human experience.

Strongly Agree	Agree	Don't Know	Disagree	Strongly Disagree

12. Religion is a very 'personal' issue.

Strongly Agree	Agree	Don't Know	Disagree	Strongly Disagree

14. Nurses should always refer patients to other agencies if they want to talk about spiritual or religious matters (eg a chaplain or a priest).

Strongly Agree	Agree	Don't Know	Disagree	Strongly Disagree

15. Most nurses are to involved in their own beliefs to be able to give patients clear advice about spiritual or religious issues.

Strongly Agree	Agree	Don't Know	Disagree	Strongly Disagree

16. Spirituality should be part of all nursing training programmes.

Strongly Agree	Agree	Don't Know	Disagree	Strongly Disagree

References

Aamodt, A.G. (1991) Ethnography and Epistemology: Generating Nursing Knowledge. In J.M. Morse (ed) *Qualitative Nursing Research*, Sage, Newbury Park, California.

Abraham, I. et al (1989) *Statistics and Quantitative Methods in Nursing:Issues and Strategies for Research and Education*, W.B. Saunders Company, Philadelphia.

Arnold, E. (1989) Burnout as a Spiritual Issue: Rediscovering Meaning in Nursing Practice. In V. Carson (ed). *Spiritual Dimensions of Nursing Practice*. W.B. Saunders Company, Philadelphia.

Arnold, E. and Boggs, K. (1989) *Interpersonal Relationships: Professional Communication Skills for Nurses*, W.B. Saunders, Philadelphia, P.A.

Ashworth, P. (1990) Hospital Chaplains - a neglected resource? *Intensive Care Nursing*:6:165-166.

Atkinson, R. et al (1981) *Introduction to Psychology*, 8th edition, Harcourt Brace Jovanovich Inc, New York.

Autton, N. (1980) The Role of the Hospital Chaplain, *Nursing Journal*:16:697.

Baly, M. (1983) Based on Trust, *Nursing Mirror*, 156, 12, 33-34.

Beattie, A. (1987) Making a Curriculum Work. In: P. Allan and M. Jolley (eds): *The Curriculum in Nursing Education*: Croom Helm, London.

Beeny, J. (1990) Spiritual Healing, *Nursing Standard*, 5:11:48-49.

Belcher, A. et al. (1989) Spirituality and Sense of Well- being in Persons with AIDS: *Holistic Nursing Practice*, 3:4:16-25.

Benner, P. (1984) *The Expert Practitioner*, Addison Wesley, New York.

Benner, P. and Wrubel, J. (1989) *The Primacy of Caring*, Addison-Wesley Publishing Company, California.

Benor, D. (1991) Spiritual Healing in Clinical Practice, *Nursing Times*, 87, 44, 35-37.

Berelson, B. (1952) *Content Analysis in Communication Research*, Free Press, Glencoe, Illinois.

Blackham, H.J. (1986) *Humanism*, Pelican, Harmondsworth.

Boehme, J. (1954) *The Confessions* ed. W. Scott Palmer, Methuen, London.

Bowers, C. (1987) Spiritual Dimensions of the Rehabilitation Journey, *Rehabilitation Nursing*, 12, 2, 90-91.

Boydel, T. (1976) *Experiential Learning*: Manchester Monograph No 5: Department of Adult and Continuing Education: University of Manchester.

Bozett, F. (1980) Practical Suggestions for the use of the audio cassette tape recorder in nursing research, *Western Journal of Nursing Research*:2:3:602-605.

Brink, P.J. and Wood, M.J. (1989) Introduction. In P.J. Brink and M.J. Wood (eds), *Advanced Design in Nursing Research*, Sage Publications, Newbury Park, California.

Brooke, V. (1987) The Spiritual Well-Being of the Elderly, *Geriatric Nursing*, 8, 4:194-195.

Brookfield, S.D. (1986) *Understanding and Facilitating Adult Learning , A Comprehensive Analysis of Principles and Effective Practices*, Open University Press, Milton Keynes.

Brookfield, S.D. (1987) *Developing Critical Thinkers: Challenging Adults to Explore Alternative Ways of Thinking and Acting*: Open University: Milton Keynes.

Bryman, A. (1988) *Quantity and Quality in Social Research*, Unwin Hyman, London.

Bugental, E. and Bugental, J. (1984) Dispiritedness - A New Perspective on a Familiar State, *Journal of Humanistic Psychology*, 24, 1, 49-67.

Bullock, A and Stallybrass, O. (eds) (1977) *The Fontana Dictionary of Modern Thought*, Fontana, London.

Burkhardt, M. and Nagai-Jacobson, M. (1985) Dealing with Spiritual Concerns of Clients in the Community, *Journal of Community Health Nursing*, 2, 4, 191-198.

Burnard, P. (1986) Picking up the pieces, *Nursing Times*, 82, 17, 37-39

Burnard, P. (1987) Towards an Epistemological Basis for Experiential Learning in Nurse Education: *Journal of Advanced Nursing*: 12, 189-193.

Burnard, P. and Chapman, C.M. (1988) *Professional and Ethical Issues in Nursing: The Code of Professional Conduct*: Wiley, Chichester.

Burnard, P. (1989) Exploring Nurse Educators' Views of Experiential Learning: a Pilot Study: *Nurse Education Today*: 9: 1: 39 -45.

Burnard, P. (1991) *A Method of Analysing Interview Transcripts in Qualitative Research*, Unpublished Paper, University of Wales, College of Medicine, Cardiff.

Burnard, P. (1988a) Searching for Meaning, *Nursing Times*, 84, 37, 34-36.

Burnard, P. (1988) The Spiritual Needs of Atheists & Agnostics, *Professional Nurse*, 4, 3:130-132.

Burnard, P. (1987) Spiritual Distress and the Nursing Response, Theoretical Consideration and Counselling Skills, *Journal of Advanced Nursing*, 12, 377-382.

Burnard, P. (1988c) Discussing Spiritual Issues with Clients, *Health Visitor*, 61, 12, 371-372.

Burnard, P. (1990) *Learning Human Skills: An Experiential Guide for Nurses*: Butterworth-Heinemann, Oxford.

Burnard, P. (1987) Self and Peer Assessment: *Senior Nurse*: 6, 5, 16-17.

Burnard, P. (1987) *A study of the ways in which experiential learning methods are used to develop interpersonal skills in nurses in Canada and the U.S.A.*: Florence Nightingale Memorial Committee: London.

Burnard, P. (1989) *Counselling Skills for Health Professionals*: Chapman and Hall, London.

Burrell, M.C. and Wright, J.S. (1983) *Some Modern Faiths*, 2nd edition, Inter Varsity Press, Leicester.

Butler, J.1726 (1970) Sermons on Human Nature. In *Fifteen Sermons*. Roberts,T.A.(ed.) SPCK, London.

Byrne, M. (1985) A Zest for Life, *Journal of Gerontological Nursing*, 11, 4, 30-33.

Campbell, A.V. (1979) Plato. Apology 3A. In *Moral Dilemmas in Medicine*. Churchill Livingstone, Edinburgh.

Carney, J. (1982) *Content Analysis*, Harper and Row, London.

Carson, V.B. (1989c) Spirituality & the Nursing Process. In V.B. Carson (ed), *Spiritual Dimensions of Nursing Practice*, W.B. Saunders Company, Philadelphia.

Carson, V.et al (1990) Hope and Spiritual Well-Being, Essentials for Living with AIDS, *Perspectives in Psychiatric Care*, 26, 2, 28-34.

Carson, V.B. (ed) (1989a) *Spiritual Dimensions of Nursing Practice*, W.B. Saunders Company, Philadelphia.

Carson, V.B. (1989b) Spiritual Development Across the Life Span. In V.B. Carson (ed), *Spiritual Dimension of Nursing Practice*, W.B. Saunders Company, Philadelphia.

Carter, D.E. (1991) Quantitative Research. In D.E. Cormack (ed) *The Research Process in Nursing*, 2nd edition, Blackwell Scientific Publications, London.

Chapman, C.R. 1977 *Sociology for Nurses*, Balliere Tindall, London.

Chase,D.P. (trans1925) Aristotle, *Nichomachean Ethics*. Dent. London.

Clifford, M. and Gruca, J. (1987) Facilitating Spiritual Care in the Rehabilitation Setting, *Rehabilitation Nursing*, 12, 6, 331-333.

Cluff, C. (1986) Spiritual Intervention Reconsidered, *Topics in Geriatric Rehabilitation*, 1:2:77-82.

Copcutt, L. (1984) Learning through Clinical Practice, *Nursing Times*, 21 Nov.43-46.

Cork, M. (1987) *Approaches to Curriculum Planning*. In B. Davis (ed): *Nursing Education: Research and Developments*: Croom Helm, London.

Couchman, W. and Dawson, J. (1990) *Nursing and Health Care Research*, Scutari Press, London.

Cox, C. (1982) Frontiers of Nursing in the 21st Century. Lessons from the Past and Present for future directions in Nursing Education, *International Journal of Nursing Studies*, 19, 1, 1-9.

Dewey J. (1916) [1966] *Democracy and Education*: Free Press: New York.

Dewey, J. (1938) [1971] *Experience and Education*: Collier Macmillan, New York.

Dobson, M. (1987) Hinderance or Help? *Senior Nurse*, 6, 6, 18-19.

Duffy, M.E. (1985) Designing Nursing Research, The Qualitative - Quantitative Debate, *Journal of Advanced Nursing*, 10, 225-232.

Edwardson, A. (1988) *3rd Year Student Nurses' Attitudes towards the Spiritual Care of their Patients*, Unpublished Dissertation, BSc (Hons) Nursing (CNAA) at Bristol Polytechnic.

Ellerhorst-Ryan, J. (1985) Selecting an Instrument to Measure Spiritual Distress, *Oncology Nursing Forum*, 12, 2, 93-99.

Ellis, D. (1980) Whatever Happened to the Spiritual Dimension? *Canadian Nurse*, 76, 2, 42-43.

English and Welsh National Boards for Nursing, Midwifery and Health Visiting: (1982) *Syllabus of Training: Part 3 (Registered Mental Nurse)*.

Ersser, S. (1991) A Search for the Therapeutic Dimensions of Nurse-Patient Interaction. In R. McMahon and A. Pearson (ed), *Nursing as a Therapy*, Chapman and Hall, London.

Ferguson, J. (1976) *An Illustrated Encyclopedia of Mysticism and the Mystery Religions*, Thames and Hudson, London.

Ferruci, P. (1928) *What We May Be*, Turnstone Press, Wellingborough.

Ferszt, G. and Taylor, P. (1988) When your Patient needs Spiritual Comfort, *Nursing*:18:4:48-49.

Field, P.A. and Morse, J. M. (1985) *Nursing Research, The Applications of Qualitative Approaches*, Chapman and Hall, London.

Forbis, P. A. (1988) Meeting Patients' Spiritual Needs, *Geriatric Nursing*:9:3:158-159.

Fox, (1975) *Encounter with Anthropology*, Penguin, Harmondsworth.

Frankl, V. (1963) *Man's Search for Meaning*, Washington Square Books, New York.

Fromant, P. (1988) Helping each other, *Nursing Times*, 84, 3, 30-32.

Frye, B. and Long, L. (1985) Spiritual Counselling Approaches Following Brain Injury, *Rehabilitation Nursing*, 10, 6, 14-15.

Garcia, J. and Maitland, S. (1983) *Walking on Water*, Virago, London.

Geertz, C. (1966) *Anthropological Approaches to Religion*, Tavistock, London.

Glaser, B.G. and Strauss, A.L. (1967) *The Discovery of Grounded Theory, Strategies for Qualitative Research*, Aldine Press, Chicago.

Goleman, D. (1972) The Buddha on meditation and states of consciousness, *Journal of Transcultural Psychology*, 14, 1. 45-62.

Goodwin, L. and Goodwin, H. (1984) Qualitative vs Quantitative Research or Qualitative and Quantitative Research, *Nursing Research*, 33, 378-380.

Granstrom, S. (1985) Spiritual Nursing Care for Oncology Patients, *Topics in Clinical Nursing*, 7, 1, 35-45.

Greaves, F. (1987) *The Nursing Curriculum: Theory and Practice*: Croom Helm: London.

Green, R. (1986) Healing & Spirituality, *The Practitioner* 230, 1087-1093.

Green, J. (1989b) Death with Dignity - Sikhism, *Nursing Times*, 85, 7, 56-57.

Green, J. (1989c) Death with Dignity - Buddhism, *Nursing Times*, 85, 9, 40-41.

Green, J. (1989a) Death with Dignity - Hinduism, *Nursing Times*, 85, 6, 50-51.

Haralambos, M. (1980) *Sociology - Themes & Perspectives*, University Tutorial Press, Slough.

Henderson, K. (1989) Dying, God & Anger - Comforting through Spiritual Care, *Journal of Psychosocial Nursing*, 27:5:17-21.

Heron, J. (1977) *Behaviour Analysis in Education and Training*: Human Potential Research Project; University of Surrey, Guildford.

Heron, J. (1982) *Education of the Affect*: Human Potential Research Project: University of Surrey, Guildford.

Heron, J. (1977) *Behavioural Analysis in Education and Training*, Human Potential Research Project, University of Surrey, Guildford.

Heron, J. (1988) *Cosmic Psychology*, Endymion Press, London

Heron, J. (1986) *Six Category Intervention Analysis*: Human Potential Research Project: University of Surrey: Guildford.

Heron, J. (1973) *Experiential Training Techniques*: Human Potential Research Project: University of Surrey, Guildford.

Heron, J. (1987) *Confessions of a Janus Brain*: Endymion Press, London.

Highfield, M. and Cason, C. (1983) Spiritual Needs of Patients. Are they recognised? *Cancer Nursing*, 6, 187-192.

Hinnels, J.R. (ed) (1984) *Dictionary of Religions*, Penguin, Harmondsworth.

Hutchinson, S. (1986) Grounded Theory, The Method. In P.L. Munhall and C.J. Oiler (eds) *Nursing Research. A Qualitative Perspective,* Appleton-Century-Crofts, Norwalk, Connecticut.

Iglehart, H. (1983) *Woman Spirit - A Guide to Women's Wisdom,* Harper & Row, San Francisco.

International Council of Nurses, I.C.N. (1973) *Code of Nursing Ethics,* I.C.N, Geneva.

Jacik, M. (1989) Spiritual Care of the Dying Adult. In V. Carson (ed) *Spiritual Dimension of Nursing Practice,* W.B. Saunders Company, Philadelphia.

James, N. (1989) Emotional Labour, Skills and Work in the Social Regulation of Feeling, *The Sociological Review,* 37:1:15-42.

Jarvis, P. (1984) *The Sociology of Adult and Continuing Education*: Croom Helm: London.

Jarvis, P. (1983) *The Theory and Practice of Adult and Continuing Education*: Croom Helm: London.

Jung, C.G. (1961) *Psychology and Religion,* Routledge and Kegan Paul, London.

Jung, C. G. (1983) *Selected Writings* Fontana, London.

Jung, C.G. (1984) *Modern Man in Search of a Soul,* Routledge, London.

Kagan, C, Evans, J., Kay, B. (1986) *A Manual of Interpersonal Skills for Nurses: An Experiential Approach*: Harper and Row, London.

Kant, I. (1985) *Fundamental Principles of the Metaphysics of Morals.* (Trans Abbott.T.K.).Library of Literal Arts, New York.

Kapleau, P. (1989) *The Wheel of Life & Death,* Rider, London.

Kierkegaard, S. (1959) *Either/Or,* Vol 1, Doubleday , New York.

Kilty, J. (1983) *Experiential Learning*: Human Potential Research Project: University of Surrey, Guildford.

Kilty, J. (1978) *Self and Peer Assessment*: Human Potential Research Project; University of Surrey, Guildford.

Kim, M. and Moritz, D. (1980) *Classification of Nursing Diagnoses*. Proceedings of the Third & Fourth National Conferences, McGraw Hill, New York.

King, V. (1989) *Women and Spirituality*, MacMillan Education Ltd, Basingstoke.

King, S. and Gregor, F. (1984) Stress and Coping in families of the critically ill, *Critical Care Nursing*, 5:4:48-51.

Kingsley, C.C.(1885) *The Water Babies*. Garland (1976) London.

Kirk, J. and Miller, M.L. (1986) *Reliability and Validity in Qualitative Research*, Sage Publications, Newbury Park, California.

Kirschenbaum, H. (1979) *On Becoming Carl Rogers*: Dell: New York.

Knowles, M. (1980) *The Modern Practice of Adult Education, From Pedagogy to Andragogy*, 2nd Edition, Follett, Chicago.

Knowles, M.S. (1978) *The Adult Learner: A Neglected Species*: Gulf: Houston, Texas.

Knowles, M.S. (1975) *Self Directed Learning*: Cambridge: New York.

Knowles M. S. and Associates (1984) *Andragogy in Action:Applying Modern Principles of Adult Learning*, Jossey Bass, San Francisco, California.

Kolb, D. (1984) *Experiential Learning*: Prentice Hall, New Jersey.

Kopp, S. (1974) *If you meet the Buddha on the road, kill him*, Sheldon Press, London.

Kubler Ross, E. (1969) *On Death & Dying*, McMillan, New York.

Labun, E. (1988) Spiritual Care, An element in nursing care planning, *Journal of Advanced Nursing*, 13, 314-320.

Lane, J. (1987) The Care of the Human Spirit, *Journal of Professional Nursing*, 3, 6, 332-337.

Law, W. (trans.) (1781) *The Works of Jacob Behmen* Volume 4, G. Robinson, London.

Leininger, M.M.(ed) (1989) *Qualitative Research Methods in Nursing*, Grune and Stratton Inc, Orlando, Florida.

Leininger, M. (1987) Importance and Uses of ethnomethods, Ethnography and ethnonursing research. In M. Cahoon (ed), *Recent Advances in Nursing*; Research Methodology, Longman Group, UK.

Ley, D. and Corless, I. (1988) Spirituality & Hospice Care, *Death Studies*, 12, 2, 101-110.

Lipson, J. (1991) The Use of Self in Ethnographic Research. In J.M. Morse (ed), *Qualitative Nursing Research*. Revised edition, Sage Publications, Newbury Park, London.

Macquarrie, J. (1972) *Existentialism*, Penguin, Harmondsworth.

Maslow, A.H. (1970) *Motivation and Personality*, 2nd edition, Harper Row, New York.

McCaffery, M. (1983) *Nursing the Patient in Pain*, Adapted for UK by Sofaer B, Harper Row, London.

McCavery, R. (1985) Spiritual care in acute illness. In O. McGilloway and F. Myco (eds), *Nursing and Spiritual Care*, Harper and Row, London.

McCracken, G. (1988) *The Long Interview*, Sage Publications Newbury Park, California.

McGilloway, O. (1985a) Religious Beliefs, Practices and Philosophies. In O. McGilloway and F. Myco (eds), *Nursing and Spiritual Care*, Harper and Row, London.

McGilloway, O. (1985b) Spiritual Care, The Potential for Healing. In O. McGilloway and F. Myco (eds), *Nursing and Spiritual Care*, Harper and Row, London.

McGilloway, O. and Myco, F.(eds) (1985) *Nursing and Spiritual Care*, Harper and Row, London.

McNeil, P. (1990) *Research Methods*, 2nd edition, Routledge, London.

Miles, R. (1987) Experiential Learning in the Curriculum. In P. Allan and M. Jolley (eds.): *The Curriculum in Nurse Education*: Croom Helm, London.

Miller, B. (1991) Caring and the Family in the Critical Care Unit, *Surgical Nurse*, 4, 4, 4-9.

Miller, J. (1985) Inspiring hope, *American Journal of Nursing*, 86, 22-25.

Molter, N. (1979) The Needs of relatives of the critically ill, A description study, *Heart and Lung*, 8, 2, 332-9.

Morrison, R. (1990) Spiritual health care and the nurse, *Nursing Standard*, 4, 36, 32-34.

Morse, J.M. (1991b) Strategies for Sampling. In J.M. Morse (ed) *Qualitative Nursing Research*, Sage Publications, Newbury Park, London.

Morse, J.M.(ed) (1991a) *Qualitative Nursing Research. A Contemporary Dialogue*, Sage Publications, Newbury Park, California.

Muldary, T. (1983) *Burnout & Health Professionals, Manifestations & Management*, Appleton & Lauge, Norwalk.

Munhall, P.L. and Oiler, C.J.(eds) (1986) *Nursing Research A Qualitative Perspective*, Appleton-Century-Crofts, Norwalk, Connecticut.

Munhall, P.L. (1989) Qualitative Designs. In P.J. Brink, and M.J. Wood (eds) *Advanced Design in Nursing Research,* Sage Publications, Newbury Park, California.

Murgatroyd, S. (1986) *Counselling and Helping:*British Psychological Society and Methuen, London.

Myco, F. (1985) The Non Believer in the Health Care Situation. In O. McGilloway and F. Myco (eds), *Nursing & Spiritual Care,* Harper and Row, London.

Neuberger, J. (1987) *Caring for Dying People of Different Faiths,* The Lisa Sainsbury Foundation Series, London.

Nye, R. (1986) *Three Psychologies,* 3rd edition, Books/ Cole Publishing Company, Monterey, California.

O'Brien, M.E. (1982) The Need for Spiritual Integrity. In H. Yura and W.B. Walsh (eds), *Human Needs 2 and the Nursing Process,* Appleton Century Crofts, Norwalk, Connecticut.

Parse, R.et al (1985) *Nursing Research. Qualitative Methods,* Brady Communications Company, Bowie, Maryland.

Pearson, A. (1991) Taking up the Challenge, The Future for Therapeutic Nursing. In R. McMahon and A. Pearson (eds), *Nursing as Therapy,* Chapman and Hall, London.

Peterson, E. (1985) The Physical... The Spiritual... Can you meet all of your patients needs?, *Journal of Gerontological Nursing,* 11, 10, 23-27.

Peterson, E. and Nelson, K. (1987) How to meet your clients' Spiritual Needs, *Journal of Psychosocial Nursing,* 25, 5, 34-39.

Piles, C. (1990) Providing Spiritual Care, *Nurse Educator,* 15, 1, 36-41.

Raichura, L. (1987) Learning by Doing: *Nursing Times*: 83, 13, 59-61.

Raths, L., Harmin, M and Simon, S. (1966) *Values and Teaching*, Merrill, Columbus, Ohio.

Ray, M.A. (1985) A Philosophical Method to Study Nursing Phenomena. In M.M. Leininger (ed) *Qualitative Research Methods in Nursing*, Grune and Stratton Inc, Orlando, Florida.

Reason, P. and Rowan, J. eds (1981) *Human Inquiry, A Sourcebook of New Paradigm Research*, John Wiley and Sons, Chichester.

Reed, P.(1987) Spirituality & Well Being in Terminally ill Hospitalised Adults, *Research in Nursing & Health*, 10, 335-344.

Riesman, D. (1950) *The Lonely Crowd*: Yale University Press: New Haven, Connecticut.

Robinson, J.A.T. (1963) *Honest to God*, SCM, London.

Rogers, C.R. (1967) *On Becoming a Person*: Constable: London.

Rogers, C.R. (1985) Towards a More Human Science of the Person: *Journal of Humanistic Psychology*: 25, 4, 7-24.

Rogers, C.R. (1984) *Freedom to Learn for the Eighties*: Merrill, Columbus, Ohio.

Rogers, C.R. (1980) *A Way of Being* , Houghton Mifflin, Boston, Mass.

Rogers, C.R. (1951) *Client-Centred Therapy*, Constable, London.

Rogers, C. (1987) Comments on the Issues of Equality in Psychotherapy, *Journal of Humanistic Psychology*, 27, 1, 27-37.

Roszak, T. (1969) *The Making of a Counter Culture: Reflections on the Technocratic Society and its Youthful Opposition*: Doubleday: New York.

Rowan, J. (1990) Spiritual Experiences in Counselling, *British Journal of Guidance & Counselling*:18:3:233-249.

Rowan, J. (1981) A Dialectical Paradigm for Research. In P. Reason and J. Rowan (eds) *Human Inquiry: A Sourcebook of New Paradigm Research*, John Wiley & Sons, Chichester.

Rumbold, (1986) *Ethics in Nursing Practice*, Balliere Tindall, London

Sampson, C. (1982) *The Neglected Ethic, Religious and Cultural Factors in the Care of Patients*, McGraw Hill, Maidenhead, Berkshire.

Sartre, J.P. (1964) *Words*, Penguin, Harmondsworth.

Sartre, J.P.(1984) *Existentialism and Humanism*. Methuen. London.

Schrock, R.(1980) A Question of Honesty in Nursing Practice. *Journal of Advanced Nursing*. 5, 2, 135-148.

Searle, J. (1983) *Intentionality, an Essay in Philosophy of Mind*, Cambridge University Press, Cambridge.

Seedhouse, D. (1988) *Ethics, The Heart of Health Care*, John Wiley & Sons, Chichester.

Shaffer, J. (1991) Spiritual Distress and Critical Illness, *Critical Care Nurse*, 11, 1, 42-45.

Shaffer, J.B.P. (1978) *Humanistic Psychology*: Prentice Hall, New Jersey.

Shaffer, J.P.B. (1978) *Humanistic Psychology*, Prentice Hall, Englewood Cliffs, New Jersey.

Shelly, J. (1982) Spiritual Care - Planning seeds of hope, *Critical Care Update*, 9, 12, 7-17.

Simmons, D. (1982) *Personal Valuing - An Introduction*, Nelson Hall, Chicago.

Simon, S, Howe, L.W. and Kirschenbaum, H. (1978) *Values Clarification*, Revised edition , A and W Visual Library, New York.

Simsen, B. (1986) The Spiritual Dimension, *Nursing Times*, November 26th:41-42.

Smith, E. (1981) The Integrated Curriculum from a Development Perspective, *Nursing Outlook*, 29, 10, 577-578.

Sodestrom, K. and Martinson, I. (1987) Patients' Spiritual Coping Strategies, A Study of Nurse & Patients Perspectives, *Oncology Nursing Forum*, 14, 2, 41-46.

Soeken, K. and Carson, V. (1986) Study Measures of Nurses' Attitudes about Providing Spiritual Care, *Health Progress*, April, 52-55.

Soeken, K. and Carson, V. (1987) Responding to the Spiritual Needs of the Chronically Ill, *Nursing Clinics of North America*, 22, 3, 603-611.

Sommer, B. and Sommer, R. (1991) *A Practical Guide to Behavioural Research, tools and techniques*, 3rd Edition, Oxford University Press, London.

Stern, P.N. (1985) Using Grounded Theory Method in Nursing Research. In M.M. Leininger (ed) *Qualitative Research Methods in Nursing*, Grune and Stratton Inc, Orlando, Florida.

Stoll, R. (1979) Guidelines for Spiritual Assessment, *American Journal of Nursing*, 9, 1574-1577.

Stoll, R. (1989a) The Essence of Spirituality. In V. Carson (ed), *Spiritual Dimensions of Nursing Practice*, W.B. Saunders Company, Philadelphia.

Storr, A. (1983) *Jung, Selected Writings*, Fontana, London.

Tart, C. (1969 *Altered States of Consciousness*, Routledge and Kegan Paul, London.

Tart, C. (ed) (1975) *Transpersonal Psychologies*, Routledge and Kegan Paul, London.

Thiroux, J.P.(1980) *Ethics, Theory and Practice* (2nd ed) Glencoe, California.

Tillich, P. (1949) [1962] *The Shaking of the Foundations*, Pelican, Harmondsworth.

Tomlinson, A. (1985) The Use of Experiential Methods in Teaching Interpersonal Skills to Nurses: In C. Kagan (ed) *Interpersonal Skills in Nursing: Research and Applications*: Kogan Page: London

Travelbee, J. (1971) *Interpersonal Aspects of Nursing*, 2nd edition, F.A. Davis Co, Philadelphia.

Treece, E.W. and Treece, J.W. (1986) *Elements of Research in Nursing*, 4th edition, The C.V. Mosby Company, St. Louis, Missouri.

Tschudin, V. (1986) *Ethics in Nursing*, Heinemann, London.

UKCC, (1987) *Project Paper 9, Project 2000 The Final Proposals*, UKCC.

United Kingdom Central Council, UKCC. (1984) *Code of Professional Conduct*, UKCC, London.

Wallis, R. (1984) *The Elementary Forms of the New Religious Life*, Routledge and Kegan Paul, London.

Weisman, A. (1979) *Coping with Cancer*, McGraw Hill, New York.

Wilson, C. (1956) *The Outsider*, Gollancz, London

Wilson, H.S. (1989) The Craft of Qualitative Analysis. In H.S. Wilson (ed) *Research in Nursing*, 2nd edition, Addison-Wesley Publishing Company Health Sciences, Redwood City, California.

Wilson-Barnett, J. (1985) *Ten Studies on Patient Care*, RCN, London.

Winkelstein, M. (1989) Spirituality and the Death of a Child. In V. Carson (ed). *Spiritual Dimensions of Nursing Practice*, W.B. Saunders Company, Philadelphia.

Yura, H. and Walsh, M. (1983) *The Nursing Process*, 4th Edition, Appleton-Century-Crofts, Norwalk, Connecticut.

Zahourek, R.P. (ed) (1988) *Relaxation and Imagery: Tools for Therapeutic Communication and Intervention*: W. B. Saunders, Philadelphia, P.A.

Bibliography

Ajzen, I. (1988) *Attitudes, Personality and Behaviour*. Open University Press, Milton Keynes.

Aroskar, M.A. (1980) Ethics of nurse-patient relationships: *Nurse Educator*: 5: 2: 18-20

Aroskar, M.A. (1980) Anatomy of an ethical dilemma: the theory, the practice. *American Journal of Nursing*: 80: 4: 658-63.

Austin R. (1978) Professionalism and the nature of nursing reward: *Journal of Advanced Nursing*: 3: 19-23.

Bailey, R. (1985) *Coping With Stress in Caring*: Blackwell, Oxford.

Baly, M. (1983) Based on trust: *Nursing Mirror*: 156:12:33-34.

Baly, M. (1980) Nursing and Social Change: 2nd Edition: *Heinemann*, London.

Baly, M. (1984) *Professional Responsibility*: 2nd Edition: Wiley, Chichester.

Banks, R., Poehler, D., Russell, R. (1984) Spirit and Human Spiritual Interaction as a Factor in Health and in Health Education. *Health Education* Aug/Sept.1984: 16-19.

Barker, P. (1989) Reflections on the philosophy of caring in mental health. *International Journal of Nursing Studies*, 26, 2, 131-141.

Barnes, H.E. (1967) *An Existential Ethics*: Knopf, New York.

Baron, R.A. and Byrne, D. (1987) *Social Psychology: Understanding Human Interaction*. 5th Edition, Allyn and Bacon, Boston.

Bartley, W.W. (1971) *Morality and Religion*: Macmillan, London

Beardshaw, V. (1981) *Conscientious Objectors at Work*: Social Audit Ltd, London.

Beck, C.M., Crittenden, B.S. and Sullivan, E.V. (eds) (1971) *Moral Education*: Toronto University Press, Toronto.

Benjamin, M. and Curtis, J. (1981) *Ethics in Nursing*: O.U.P. New York.

Benner, P. (1984) *From Novice to Expert: Excellence and Power in Clinical Nursing Practice*. Addison-Wesley, Menlo Park, California.

Benner, P. and Wrubel, J. (1989) *The Primacy of Caring: Stress and Coping in Health and Illness*: Addison Wesley, Menlo Park.

Bergman, R. (1976) Evolving ethical concepts for nursing: *International Nursing Review*: 23: 4: 116-17.

Berry, C. (1987) *The Rites of Life: Christians and Bio-Medical Decision Making*: Hodder and Stoughton, London.

Blackham, H.J. (1968) *Humanism*: Pelican, Harmondsworth.

Blomquist, C., Veatch, R.M. and Fenner, D. (1975) The teaching of medical ethics: *Journal of Medical Ethics*: 1: 2: 96-103.

Bok, S. (1980) Lying: Moral Choice in Public and Private Life: *Quartet*, London.

Bontell, K & Bozett, F. (1990) Nurses' Assessment of Patients' Spiritual; Continuing Education Implications. *The Journal of Continuing Education in Nursing* 21: 4: 172-176.

British Medical Association (1980) *Handbook of Medical Ethics*: B.M.A., London.

Broad, C.D. (1930) *Five Types of Ethical Theory*: Routledge and Kegan Paul: London.

Brody, J.K. (1988) Virtue ethics, caring and nursing. *Scholarly Inquiry for Nursing Practice: An International Journal*, 2, 2, 87-96.

Brown, L. (1986) The experience of care: patient perspectives. *Topics in Clinical Nursing*, 8, 2, 56-62.

Bruner, L. (1984) The Spiritual Dimension of Holistic Care. *Imprint* 4: 44-45.

Bryan, J.H. and Test, M.A. (1967) Models and helping: naturalistic studies in aiding behaviour. *Journal of Personality and Social Psychology*, 6, 4, 400-407.

Buber, M. (1937) *I and Thou*: T.and T. Clark: Edinburgh.

Bunzl, M: A note on nursing ethics in the U.S.A. *Journal of Medical Ethics*: 1: 4: 184.

Burkhardt, M. (1989) Spirituality: An analysis of the Concept. *Holistic Nursing Practice* 3, 69-77.

Burnard, P. (1987) Spiritual distress and the nursing response: theoretical considerations and counselling skills: *Journal of Advanced Nursing*:12: 377-382.

Campbell, A.V. (1984) *Moderated Love*: S.P.C.K. London.

Campbell, A.V. and Higgs, R. (1982) *In that Case*: Darton, Longman and Todd, London.

Campbell, A.V. (1984) *Moral Dilemmas in Medicine*: 3rd Edition: Churchill Livingstone, Edinburgh.

Campbell, A. (1985) *Paid to Care: the Limits of Professionalism in Pastoral Care*. SPCK, London.

Carper, B.A. (1979) The ethics of caring. *Advances in Nursing Science*, 1, 3, 11-19.

Cash, K. (1990) Nursing models and the idea of nursing. *International Journal of Nursing Studies*, 27, 3, 249-256.

Chapman, C.M. (1977) Concepts of Professionalism: *Journal of Advanced Nursing*: 2: 51-55.

Christie, R.J. and Hoffmaster, C.B. (1986) *Ethical Issues in Family Medicine*: Oxford University Press, New York.

Churchill, L. (1977) Ethical issues of a profession in transition: *American Journal of Nursing*: 77: 5: 873-875.

Cook, J. (1987) *Whose Health is it Anyway?*: New English Library, Sevenoaks, Kent.

Cox, C. (1979) Who cares? Nursing and Sociology: the development of a symbiotic relationship: *Journal of Advanced Nursing*: 4: 237-252.

Dalley, G. (1988) *Ideologies of Caring: Rethinking Community and Collectivism*. Macmillan, London.

Daniels, V. and Horowitz, L.J. (1984) *Being and Caring: A Psychology for Living*: 2nd Edition: Mayfield, Mountain View, California.

Dass, R. & Gorman, P. (1985) *How Can I Help? Emotional support and spiritual inspiration for those who care for others*. London: Rider.

Davis, H. and Fallowfield, L. (eds) (1991) *Counselling and Communication in Health Care*. Wiley, Chichester.

Davis, A.J. and Aroskar, M.A. (1983) *Ethical Dilemmas and Nursing Practice*: Appleton-Century-Crofts: Norwalk, Connecticut.

Dickinson, C. (1975) The Search for Spiritual Meaning. *American Journal of Nursing* 75: 10: 1789-1794.

Downie, R.S. and Calman, K.C. (1987) *Healthy Respect: Ethics in Health Care*: Faber and Faber, London.

Doxiadis, S. (ed) (1987) *Ethical Dilemmas in Health Promotion*: Wiley, Chichester.

Dugan, D. (1987) Death and Dying. Emotional, Spiritual and Ethical Support for Patient and families. *Journal of Psychosocial Nursing* 1987: 25: 7: 21-29.

Duncan, A.S., Dunstan, G.R. and Welbourne, R.B. (1981) *Dictionary of Medical Ethics* 2nd Edition: Darton, Longman and Todd, London.

Dunlop, M.J. (1986) Is a science of caring possible? *Journal of Advanced Nursing*: 11:661-670.

Dunstan, G.R. and Seller, M.J. (eds) (1983) *Consent in Medicine*: King Edward's Hospital Fund, London.

Dunstan, G.R. (1974) *The Artifice of Ethics*: SCM, London.

Durkheim, E. (1961) *Moral Education*: The Free Press, Glencoe, Ill.

Ededel, A. (1955) *Ethical Judgement*: The Free Press: Glencoe, New York.

Ellis, C. (1987) Teaching Spiritual Care of Patients. *Journal of Nursing Staff Development* 3: 1: 43-44.

Ferguson, M. and Turner, V. (1976) The dilemma of professionalism and Nursing Organisation: *Nursing Mirror*: 16th December.

Field, D. (1984) 'We didn't want him to die on his own'-Nurses' accounts of nursing dying patients. *Journal of Advanced Nursing*, 9, 59-70.

Finch, J. and Groves, D. (eds) (1983) *A Labour of Love: Women, Work and Caring*. Routledge and Kegan Paul , London.

Fletcher, J. (1955) *Morals and Medicine*: Gollancz, London.

Forrest, D. (1989) The experience of caring. *Journal of Advanced Nursing*, 14, 815-823.

Fox, F.E. 1983 The Spiritual Core of Experiential Education: *Journal of Experiential Education*: 16: 1: 3 - 6.

Francis, B. (1990) Patient Care-The Spiritual Dimension. *Advancing Clinical Care*: 5: 5: 7-8.

Frankena, W.K. (1973) *Ethics*: Prentice Hall, Englewood Cliffs, New Jersey.

Friedson, E. (1976) The Future of Professionalism. In Stacey et al, (1977) *Health and the Division of Labour*: Croom Helm, London.

Fromm E. (1976) *To Have or To Be?* Abacus, London.

Gardner, R.F.R. (1977) *By What Standard?*: Christian Medical Federation , London.

Gillon, R. (1986) *Philosophical Medical Ethics*: Wiley, Chichester.

Goodman, C. (1986) Research on the informal carer: a selected literature review. *Journal of Advanced Nursing*, 11, 705-712.

Griffin, A.P. (1983) A philosophical analysis of caring in nursing: *Journal of Advanced Nursing*: 8: 289-295.

Hall, J. (1990) Towards a psychology of caring. *British Journal of Clinical Psychology*, 29, 129-144.

Haring, B. (1974) *Medical Ethics*: St Paul Publications, Slough.

Harmin, M, Kirschenbaum, H. and Simon, S. (1973) *Clarifying Values Through Subject Matter*: Winston Press, Minneapolis.

Harris, J. (1986) *The Value of Life: An introduction to medical ethics*: Routledge and Kegan Paul, London.

Harrison, L.L. (1990) Maintaining the ethic of caring in nursing. *Journal of Advanced Nursing*, 15, 125-127.

Hendricks, G. and Fadiman, J. (eds) 1976 *Transpersonal Education: a Curriculum for Feeling and Being*: Prentice Hall, Englewood Cliffs, New Jersey.

Henley, A. (1982) *Asians in Britain. Caring for Muslims and their Families. Religious Aspects of Care*. London: DHSS/Kings Fund

Hirst, P.H. (1974) *Moral Education in a Secular Society*: University of London Press, London.

Horan, F. and Jackson, V. (1984) Abortion: who decides?: *Nursing Times*: 80: 10: 16-18.

Hoy, R. and Robbins, (1979) *The Profession of Nursing*: McGraw Hill, London.

Hudson, W.D. (1970) *Modern Moral Philosophy*: Macmillan, London.

Hurding, R.F. (1985) *Roots and Shoots: a guide to counselling and psychotherapy*. Hodder and Stoughton, London.

Hyde, A. (1976) The phenomenon of caring: *Nursing Research Report*: 11:3: 2 and 19.

Illich, I. (1975) *Medical Nemesis: the Expropriation of Health,* Calder and Boyars, London.

Jackson, D.M. (1972) *Professional Ethics: Who makes the rules?*: C.M.F. Publications, London.

Jameton, A. (1984) *Nursing Practice: the Ethical Issues*: Prentice Hall, New Jersey.

Jarvis, P. (1983) Religiosity: a theoretical analysis of the human response to the problem of meaning: Institute for the study of Worship and Religious Architecture, *Research Bulletin*: 51-66.

Jarvis, P. (1987) Meaningful and Meaningless Experience: Towards an Understanding of Learning From Life: *Adult Education Quarterly*: 37: 3.

Johnson, M. (1983) Ethics in nurse education: a comment: *Nurse Education Today*: 3: 58-59.

Jupe, M. (1987) Ethics and Nursing Practice: *Senior Nurse*: 7: 3: 49-51.

Keenan, B. (1992) *An Evil Cradling*. London: Hutchinson.

Kemp, J. (1970) *Ethical Naturalism*. Macmillan, London.

Kennedy, I. (1981) *Unmasking Medicine*. Allen and Unwin, London.

Kirschenbaum, H. (1977) *Advanced Values Clarification*: University Associates, La Jolla, California.

Kitson, A.L. (1987) A comparative analysis of lay caring and professional caring relationships: *International Journal of Nursing Studies*: 24: 2: 155-165.

Kleinig, J. (1985) *Ethical Issues in Psychosurgery*: Allen and Unwin, London.

Kleinman, A. (1988) *The Illness Narratives: Suffering, Healing and the Human Condition*. Basic Books, New York.

Knight, M. and Field, D. (1981) Silent conspiracy: coping with dying cancer patients on acute surgical wards. *Journal of Advanced Nursing*, 6, 221-229.

Larson, P.J. (1984) Important nurse caring behaviours perceived by patients with cancer. *Oncology Nursing Forum*, 11, 6, 46-50.

Leininger, M.M. (1988) History, issues, and trends in the discovery and uses of care in nursing. In: M.M. Leininger (ed) *Care: Discovery and Uses in Clinical and Community Nursing*. Wayne State University Press, Detroit, pp.11-28.

Leininger, M.M. (1981) The phenomenon of caring: importance, research questions and theoretical considerations. In: M.M. Leininger (ed) *Caring: an Essential Human Need*. Charles B. Slack, New Jersey, pp.3-15.

Levine, S. (1986) *Who Dies? An investigation of conscious living and conscious dying*. Bath: Gateway Books.

Levine, M. (1977) Ethics: nursing ethics and the ethical nurse: *American Journal of Nursing*: 77 ; 5 ; 845-849.

Lewis, D. (1987) All in Good Faith. *Nursing Times* March 18: 40-43.

Llewelyn, S.P. (1989) Caring: the cost to nurses and relatives. In: A.K. Broome (ed) *Health Psychology: Processes and Applications*. Chapman and Hall, London, pp.114 - 129.

Males, J. & Boswell, C. (1990) Spiritual Needs of People with a Mental Handicap. *Nursing Standard*:4: 48: 35-37.

McFarlane, J. (1976) A charter for caring. *Journal of Advanced Nursing*, 1, 187- 196.

McGilloway, F. & Donnelly, L. (1977) Religion and Patient Care: the functionalist approach. *Journal of Advanced Nursing* 2: 3-13.

McGilloway, O. and Myco, F (eds) 1985 *Nursing and Spiritual Care*: Harper and Row, London.

McGlone, M. (1990) Healing the Spirit. *Holistic Nursing Practice* July: 4: 4: 77-84.

Merritt, J. (1991) Hope outside the cancer ward. *Sunday Observer* July 14: 50.

Meyers, D.W. (1970) *The Human Body and the Law*: Edinburgh University Press, Edinburgh.

Morris, C. (1956) *Varieties of Human Value*: University of Chicago Press, Chicago.

Morrison, P. (1988) Nurses' perceptions of caring. *Nursing Times*, 84, 9, 51.

Morrison, R. (1989) Spiritual Health Care and the Nurse. *Nursing Standard*: 4: 13: 28-29.

Morrison, P. (1991) The caring attitude in nursing practice: a repertory grid study of trained nurses' perceptions. *Nurse Education Today*, 11, 3-12.

Morrison, P. (1989) Nursing and caring: a personal construct theory study of some nurses' self-perceptions. *Journal of Advanced Nursing*, 14, 421-426.

Morrison, P. and Burnard, P. (1991) *Caring and Communicating: The Interpersonal Relationship in Nursing*. Macmillan, London.

Nagai-Jacobson, M. & Burkchardt, M. (1989) Spirituality: Cornerstone of holistic nursing practice. *Holistic Nursing Practice*: 3: 3: 18-26.

Nehring, V. and Geach, B. (1973) Patients' evaluation of their care: why they don't complain. *Nursing Outlook*, 21, 5, 317-321.

Neuberger, J. (1987) *Caring for People of Different Faiths*: Austin Cornish, London.

Newman, M. (1989) The spirit of nursing. *Holistic Nursing Practice* May: 3: 3: 1-6.

Nightingale, F. (1974) *Notes on Nursing: what it is and what it is not*: New Edition: Blackie, London.

Papper, S. (1983) *Doing Right: Everyday Medical Ethics*: Little Brown, Boston.

Partridge, K.B. (1978) Nursing values in a changing society: *Nursing Outlook*: 26: 6: 356-360.

Paterson, J.G. and Zderad, L.T. (1988) *Humanistic Nursing*. National League for Nursing, New York.

Patka, F. (ed) (1972) *Existential Thinkers and Thought*: Citadel Press, Secaucus, New Jersey.

Paton, H.J. (1969) *The Moral Law: Kant's Groundwork of the Metaphysics of Morals*: Hutchinson, London.

Phillips, M. and Dawson, J. (1985) *Doctors' Dilemmas: Medical Ethics and Contemporary Science*: Harvester Press, Brighton, Sussex.

Ramsey, P. (1970) *The Patient as Person: Explorations in Medical Ethics*: Yale University press, New Haven, Connecticut.

Ramsey, P. (1965) *Deeds and Rules in Christian Ethics*: Cambridge University Press, Cambridge.

Ramsey, P. (1978) *Ethics at the Edges of Life: Medical and Legal Intersections*: Yale University Press, New Haven, Connecticut.

Ray, M.A. (1981) A study of caring within an institutional culture. *Dissertation Abstracts International*, 42, 6, 2310-b.

Ray, M.A. (1987) Technological caring: a new model in critical care. *Dimensions of Critical Care Nursing*, 6, 3, 166-173.

Ray, M.A. (1981) A philosophical analysis of caring within nursing. In: M.M. Leininger (ed) *Caring: an Essential Human Need*. Charles B. Slack, New Jersey, pp.25-36.

Reed, P. (1986) Religiousness among Terminally Ill and Healthy Adults. *Research in Nursing and Health* 9: 35-41.

Reich, W.T. (1978) *Encyclopedia of Bioethics*: 4 Volumes: Macmillan, London.

Reiser, S.J., Dyck, A.J. and Curran, W.T. (1977) *Ethics in Medicine*, M.I.T. Press, Boston.

Rew, L. (1989) In tuition: Nursing knowledge and the spiritual dimension of persons. *Holistic Nursing Practice* May: 3: 3: 56-68.

Riemen, D. (1986) The essential structure of a caring interaction: doing phenomenology. In: P.L. Munhall, and Oiler, C.J. (eds) *Nursing Research: a Qualitative Perspective*. Appleton-Century-Crofts, Norwalk, Connecticut, 85-108.

Roach, Sr. M.S. (1987) *The Human Act of Caring: a Blueprint for the Health Professions*. Canadian Hospital Association, Ottawa, Ontario.

Roach, M.S. (1984) *Caring, the Human Mode of Being, Implications for Nursing*: University of Toronto.

Rogers, C.R. (1977) *On Personal Power*: Constable, London.

Rumbold, G. (1986) *Ethics in Nursing Practice*: Balliere Tindall, London.

Samarel, N. (1989) Caring for the living and the dying: a study of role transition. *International Journal of Nursing Studies*, 26, 4, 313-326.

Sampson, C. (1982) *The Neglected ethic: Religious and Cultural Factors in the Care of Patients*: McGraw Hill, London.

Sarason, S.B. (1985) *Caring and Compassion in Clinical Practice*. Jossey-Bass, London.

Sartre, J-P. (1973) *Existentialism and Humanism*: Translated P. Mairet: Methuen, London.

Schrock, R. (1980) A Question of Honesty in Nursing Practice: *Journal of Advanced Nursing*: 5: 2; 135-148.

Schulman, E.D. (1982) *Intervention in Human Services: A Guide to Skills and Knowledge*: 3rd Edition: C.V. Mosby: St Louis, Toronto.

Scorer, G. and Wing, A. (eds) (1979) *Decision Making in Medicine: the practice of its ethics*: Arnold, London.

Scott, R. (1981) *The Body as Property*: Viking Press, London.

Scrivenger, M. (1987) Ethics, Etiquette and the Law: *Nursing Times*: 83: 42: 28-29.

Sedgwick, P. (1982) *Psycho Politics* Pluto Press, London.

Sieghart, P. (1985) Professions as the conscience of society: *Journal of Medical Ethics*: 11: 3: 117-122.

Simmons, D. (1982) *Personal Valuing: an Introduction*: Helson Hall, Chicago.

Simon, S.B., Howe, L.W. and Kirschenbaum, H. (1978) *Values Clarification: A Handbook of Practical Strategies for Teachers and Students*: A and W. Visual Library, New York.

Simsen, B. (1988) Nursing the spirit. *Nursing Times* 14.9.88: 31-33.

Stacey, M. (1988) *The Sociology of Health and Healing: A Textbook*. Unwin Hyman, London.

Steele, S.M. and Harmon, V.M. (1983) *Values Clarification in Nursing*: 2nd Edition: Appleton-Century-Crofts: Norwalk, Connecticut.

Stephenson, M. and Moran, L. (1987) The dilemma of ethics: *Senior Nurse*: 7:3: 47-48.

Stuart, E. et al (1989) Spirituality in Health and Healing: A Clinical Program. *Holistic Nursing Practice* 3: 3: 35-46.

Styles, M.M. (1982) *On Nursing: Towards a new endowment*: C.V. Mosby: St Louis.

Tate, .B.L. (1977) *The Nurses Dilemma: Ethical Considerations in Nursing Practice*: I.C.N. Code, Geneva.

Thiroux, J.P. (1980) *Ethics, Theory and Practice*: 2nd Edition: Glencoe Publishing: Encino, California.

Thompson, I.A., Melia, K. and Boyd, K. (1983) *Nursing Ethics*: Churchill Livingstone, Edinburgh.

Thompson, I.,E. et al (1981) Research Ethical Committees in Scotland: *British Medical Journal*: 282: 718-720.

Thomson, W.A.R. (1977) *A Dictionary of Medical Ethics and Practice*: Wright, Bristol.

Thorne, B. (1990) Spiritual Dimensions in Counselling. Editors Introduction. *British Journal of Guidance and Counselling* 18: 3: 225-233.

Tillich, P. (1963) *Morality and Beyond*: Harper and Row, London.

Toulmin, S. (1958) *The Place of Reason in Ethics*: Cambridge University Press, Cambridge.

Townesend, P. and Davidson, N. (1982) *Inequalities in Health*: Penguin, Harmondsworth.

Trower, P., O'Mahony, J.M. and Dryden, W. (1982) Cognitive aspects of social failure: Some implications for social skills training: *British Journal of Guidance and Counselling*: 10, 176 - 184.

Tschudin, V. (1986) *Ethics in Nursing: the Caring Relationship*: Heinemann, London.

Van Hooft, S. (1987) Caring and professional commitment. *The Australian Journal of Advanced Nursing*, 4, 4, 29-38.

Veatch, R.M. (1977) *Case Studies in Medical Ethics*: Harvard University Press, Cambridge, Mass.

Veness, D. (1990) Spirituality and Counselling: a view from the other side. *British Journal of Guidance and Counselling* 18: 3: 250-260.

Warnock, M. (1970) *Existentialism*: Oxford University Press, London.

Watson, J. (1985) *Nursing: Human Science and Human Care: A theory of nursing*: Appleton-Century-Crofts: Norwalk, Connecticut.

Watson, J. (1979) *Nursing: The Philosophy and Science of Caring*: Little, Brown and Co, New York.

Williams, B. (1976) *Morality: An Introduction to Ethics*: Cambridge University Press, Cambridge.

Wright, D. (1971) *The Psychology of Moral Behaviour*: Penguin, Harmondsworth.

Index